Storytelling for Life

Storytelling
for Life

Why Stories Matter
and Ways of Telling Them

Josie Felce

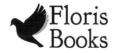 Floris
Books

First published in 2012 by Floris Books
Second printing 2022

© 2012 Josie Felce

British Library CIP Data available
ISBN 978-086315-923-7

To the next generation of storytellers:
may they rest their backs on the wisdom of ancient stories
and have the insight to create new ones.

Acknowledgements

Thanks to: Steve Killick, Cynthia Morgan and Martin Hardiman for reading through and advising me on early drafts of the book, and to Sally Polson of Floris Books for restructuring it and encouraging me to fulfil its aim; Sue Harker for going through the Steiner story curriculum on a bus through Spain; Annabel Hollis for sharing her responses to key adult stories; Sheila McCartney for telling me the story of *The Prince and the Ring*; Kelvin Hall for his work on personal stories; Dennis Gould for his infectious enthusiasm for words and books; George Richards for computer help; and Christine Felce for helpful flower remedies. Apologies to anyone I have quoted but not named.

Quotations from Rudolf Meyer's *The Wisdom of Fairy Tales* are reproduced with kind permission from Floris Books. Quotations from *The Sense of Being Stared At and Other Aspects of the Extended Mind* by Rupert Sheldrake, published by Hutchinson, are reprinted by kind permission of The Random House Group Limited.

Contents

List of stories   11
Preface   13

1. The importance of storytelling   15
2. What is a fairy tale?   27
3. Stories for transformation and healing   35
4. Teller and listener   54
5. Storytelling skills   60
6. Personal stories   79
7. Ages and stages: stories in education   86
8. Adults: the ongoing journey   102
9. An exercise of the spirit   119

Bibliography   132
    Story Sources   134
    Useful websites   135

Be it heard
Or be it told,
A story is a gift
Worth more than gold.

List of Stories

Tom Who Was Scared of the Dark 16
Seventeen Camels 22
Truth and Story 26
Maybe, Maybe Not 38
The Prince and the Ring 40
A New Dawn 41
The Man who was Sad 42
The Tree at the Crossroads 45
The Cracked Pot 45
The Hollow in the Stone 46
How an African Hunts 47
The Rabbi's Gift 48
The Girl with Big Feet 51
The Listener 59
The Three Golden Eggs (1) 64
The Three Golden Eggs (2) 67
Hatching the Golden Egg 83
The Black Prince 98
Rangada 111
The King Who was Miserable 113
Jumping Mouse 121
The Secret of Creation 126

Preface

Over the last twenty years, storytelling in Britain has seen a revival. New storytellers started storytelling clubs, long-practiced ones came out into public view, and storytelling festivals were established from Edinburgh to Cardiff, Norwich to Cape Clear Island. Storytelling is the oldest form of education and public performance; it has an eternal character. It is kept alive by our need to tell stories to children, neighbours and strangers; the human desire for self-discovery; and the curiosity we feel about the history and mythology of a place, country or culture.

Why do I want to write *about* storytelling, and not just keep telling the stories? Surely telling stories to an audience, whether of children or adults, is like theatre: a shared moment there and then, with each person taking away their own impressions and meaning? But what *do* people take away with them? Why do I tell stories? Why these particular stories? What do I, as the storyteller, take away? How can telling traditional stories help us in our modern lives?

I have been connected to Steiner-Waldorf education for over a decade. I have learnt a great deal from its underlying philosophy (called 'anthroposophy') and from its abundant use of stories throughout the stages of children's development. Many teachers and parents do not come across the Steiner approach, in part because it is classed as private education and the schools and nurseries are normally fee paying. I want to prise open this gilded cage and make available to a wider group of people an understanding that encourages imaginative yet reasoned telling of stories throughout school years, and beyond. This book is for anyone interested in the practice of storytelling, particularly parents, teachers, therapists and storytellers.

World mythology is vast, and I can only draw on the stories I am familiar with. While telling stories to adults and children over the past two decades, I have discovered treasures that I would like to share with the next generation of storytellers.

I also include in this book suggestions on how to tell stories, discussion of their healing and transforming possibilities and an exploration of how our everyday conversational storytelling creates the future.

Your comments on the ideas in this book are welcome. My contact details can be found at www.storymagic.co.uk.

Josie Felce, 2012

1. The importance of storytelling

Story water

A story is like water
that you heat for your bath.

It takes messages between the fire
and your skin. It lets them meet,
and it cleans you!

RUMI

When children jump up and down with unbridled joy, adults are filled with delight and everyone is energised with life. In contrast to the sugary pleasure of sweets, stories offer nourishment of the heart and soul.

When I tell stories in primary schools, the children call out to me at break-time, 'Storyteller, storyteller, are you coming again tomorrow?' They are not really calling out to me, but for the experience of having heard a story that moves them, an experience in which they felt involved, alive, enriched. Some older teachers comment, 'We used to start our lessons with stories in the old days.' Good teachers captivate their students to engage them in the lesson; what better way than with a story?

Very recently I was in a large bookshop telling stories at half-term, when a five-year-old boy recognised me as the storyteller who had visited his school four months previously. 'I am still dreaming of Tom and the dragon that got smaller and smaller,' he told me. I remembered that I had told his class the story 'Tom Who Was

Scared of the Dark'. Until that moment I had underestimated the power of telling such stories to young children.

Tom Who Was Scared of the Dark

Once there was a boy called Tom who was scared of the dark. When it was time for bed he would shiver as he went up the creaking old stairs to his bedroom, imagining all sorts of wild things following him.

One spring morning as he walked over the fields he saw a hare stuck in a thicket. The thorny bush held the creature so it could go neither forwards nor backwards. Tom saw that it would die unless he did something to help it. He got out his pocket knife and carefully cut through the prickly stems. To his surprise, the hare did not run away but turned and spoke to him,

'Thank you for saving my life. I will grant you one wish.'

'One wish,' said Tom, 'well, I wish I wasn't scared of the dark.'

'Then look at the moon and think of me, and all your fears will fade into the night,' said the hare, before it leapt away over the field.

When winter came, the evenings were long and dark. Tom's mother would give him a candle in a candle holder to take upstairs to bed. One evening the flickering flame threw shadows on the walls and he was glad to get to bed and pull the blankets up over his face. As he began to relax, his head came out of the blankets and a slimy cold thing dropped onto his face! He sat up in bed. A full moon came out from behind the clouds and he remembered the hare and his promise. All the fear left him. He said to himself, 'If something has fallen onto my face, then I must take it off.' He peeled the slimy thing off his face and saw that it was a spider's web. It looked so beautiful in the moonlight that he put it on his bedside table so he could look at it again in the morning.

The following night as he climbed the stairs to bed, the wind rattled the windows in their frames and the candle sent huge flickering shadows onto the walls. He jumped into bed, blew out the candle and hid under the bedclothes. But as he felt sleepy, his head once again slid out onto the pillow. A sharp *screech-scratch, screech-scratch* at the window made him sit up in bed. He thought it might be some enormous bird trying to break the windowpane. Then he saw the moon and remembered the hare, and that fear left him.

He thought, 'If there is something scratching the other side of the window, I must open it, and find out what it is.' He opened the window and found a branch of the apple tree was scraping against the windowpane. He broke off the twig, shut the window and went soundly to sleep.

The next night a storm was raging. Every door and window rattled in its frame, and even the roof of the house sounded as if it was about to fly off. As he went upstairs with his candlestick, the flame made such shadows that his skin came up in goose pimples.

He got into bed and buried himself in the blankets. Just as he was drifting off to sleep, he heard it. *Bang, crash, rattle, rattle, rattle.* It sounded like a giant monster coming down the garden path. Just then, the moon appeared from behind the clouds, and Tom thought of the hare and all his fear left him.

'If there is something coming down the garden path, then I must go and see what it is,' he thought. He then did something he had never done before. He got out of bed, pulled on his clothes, went downstairs and put on his boots and jacket. He opened the back door and went outside into the cold, stormy night. The dreadful noise was not coming from the front path but from the chicken run in the garden. He saw that the henhouse door had come unfastened and the door was banging in the wind. He shut the door and fastened it with a piece of wire. He went back to bed and slept until morning.

He told his mother what had happened in the night. She was amazed.

'Tom, if you hadn't shut the henhouse door, the fox would have got in and taken them. You are the bravest boy in the whole wide world!'

Tom seemed to grow two inches taller as he sat at breakfast, he was so proud of himself. Now he wanted to tell his friends. As soon as he could, he went off out of the house. At the end of the road, several of his friends were waiting for him. Tom called,

'Hey, I'm the bravest boy in the whole wide world. My mother says so!'

'Well, if that's so,' said one, 'then maybe you can go and catch the dragon that has appeared on top of the hill.'

Tom looked up to the top of the hill. There was a huge green dragon, its tail swishing from side to side, breathing flames into the sky.

'That dragon is dangerous,' said another friend. 'It will come down here and eat up anything or anyone it can find, maybe you and I.'

Tom cut a long stout stick from the hedge and began to walk up the hill. He walked and walked. It seemed the longer he walked the further away the top of the hill became. He kept his eye on the dragon and noticed that the nearer he grew to it, the smaller it seemed to get. When he finally got to the summit of the hill, he looked down and saw the dragon was no bigger than a frog. He bent down, picked it up and put it in his pocket. Coming down the hill was much quicker. His friends were there waiting.

'Have you caught the dragon?' they asked. Tom reached into his pocket and pulled it out.

'Here it is,' he said. His friends all looked at it.

'Is that what we were all scared of?' they asked. Tom knew all about fear now.

He replied, 'Yes. The nearer you go to the thing you are scared of, the smaller it gets.'

A story is a feast offered to listeners: an invitation to taste something that will cure the thirst and hunger of a place deep within. A story creates a world where anyone who enters can safely experience new feelings and perceptions, where metaphor can allow an alternative experience. Language and mythology are part of the way we think and feel. They resist scientific attempts to reduce them and categorise them into neat compartments. In stories, the impossible becomes possible: colours appear in a grey reality, active interest is returned to boring repetitive daily tasks. Stories feed our imaginations and nourish our deep psyche.

There is a great difference between telling and reading a story, for both adults and children. It is wonderful to share a written story or a picture book with a child in a loving gesture. But reading a story to a class of children is another matter – if you are a teacher you will have experienced this. It may work for a while, but the reader has their eyes on the written page and not on the children, and the words can become deadening or unsuitable and the voice monotonous.

In telling a story, as distinct from reading, the teller looks at the children and adapts the story to their level of understanding and their needs. In live storytelling the imagination of the teller is opened so that the words can come from a deeper place within their psyche. Telling stories rather than reading them develops the imagination of both teller and listener, forming a close connection between them. The active intention of the teller is essential if the story's meaning is to be communicated. When a narrator puts feeling and expression into a story they love, this is picked up by children. If the story is delivered flatly without reaching out to meet the level or interest of the children, then it loses much of its power.

Without stories of the past, we are disconnected from our inheritance and our ancestors' witty and wise instructions. 'When we forget the truths that gave courage and strength to the ancestors of all races and creeds, we have lost ourselves and our roots,' says the wisdom-keeper Jamie Sams. (Sams, 1994) Our sense of identity and inner security is built on our connection to our parents, grandparents and guardians, who pass their personal stories to us.

Children develop emotional intelligence by being immersed in stories that deal with the challenges they face in growing up: a mere mouse can help a ferocious lion by biting through the net trapping him; a small but crafty person overcomes a powerful giant; a good-hearted hero/heroine can survive abusive treatment, find wise helpers and achieve sovereignty. A story can be a wise invisible friend, giving courage, faith and hope to its carrier, as well as to listeners.

The importance of telling stories to children is recognised in modern psychology: archetypal characters help overcome infantile polarities of love and hate. Hearing their extreme feelings personified into characters such as witches, wizards, ogres, giants, powerful queens and kings, while held in loving security by their parents, helps young children develop a balanced personality, able to cope with their own feelings of anger, rage and fear. (Skynner and Cleese, 1983)

Stories can help neglected and abused children in unexpected ways. Therapist Jean Shinoda Bolen reports that neglected and abused children who had heard stories drew solace from an inner source and so did not identify with their oppressors and did not grow up repeating their abuse. Instead they drew wisdom from beyond their years, surviving an abusive childhood without loss of soul. (Bolen, 2002)

New initiatives use storytelling to teach 'emotional literacy' in schools. The UK government's Social and Emotional Aspects of Learning (SEAL) programme lists five domains of emotional intelligence: self-awareness, managing emotions, motivation, empathy and social competence. (These domains have been taken from the writing of Daniel Goleman, whose book *Emotional*

Intelligence has been highly influential.) Choosing and creating stories helps children develop skills in understanding and managing feelings, and encourages interaction. These activities, along with telling appropriate stories in morning circle time in the classroom, have effects clearly documented by two pioneers in this field. Taffy Thomas, the first UK Storytelling Laureate, and Steve Killick, a Consultant Clinical Psychologist and also a storyteller, have collaborated in the book *Telling Tales: Storytelling as Emotional Literacy*. It explains their theory of the emotional benefits of storytelling, gives practical guidelines for beginning storytelling, and contains potent stories. (Thomas and Killick, 2007)

In Steiner-Waldorf schools, stories are part of the curriculum that helps to unfold the growing child in a specific way. Steiner curriculum is grounded in anthroposophy, Rudolph Steiner's philosophy, such that education follows the evolution of human thought through the child's development into an adult. Steiner looked at human development in a spiritual way rather than being concerned with what might be considered useful or convenient. At the turn of the nineteenth century, practicality was paramount. Technological inventions were lauded for their utility: surfaced roads, bridges, trains, cars, aeroplanes and light bulbs were new and glorious. Steiner, in contrast, looked at human origins and created a spiritual science for education, which branched into gardening, farming, movement (eurythmy), drawing (form drawing) and cosmology. Anthroposophy recognises the divine origin of mankind; we are all souls developing through many lifetimes. It is a philosophy that covers vast areas of knowledge, so here I will focus on the use of stories in education.

As a child grows up, their consciousness evolves in a parallel way to the historical evolution of human civilisations. Thus, giving very ancient stories to very young children and then, as they grow and learn, giving stories following the development of civilisations until modern times, enables the mind and soul to develop easily and fully. Children then have the best education for freedom in their adult life. Freedom means being able to choose independently using personal intuition rather than being swayed by the fashion of the day or other imposed expectations.

At the beginning of a new topic, a Steiner teacher will tell a story that illuminates the material to come. Building simple structures could be introduced to nine year olds with 'The Three Little Pigs'. Fractions could be accompanied by stories that incorporate arithmetic, such as the Egyptian tale 'Seventeen Camels'. Geology demands some creation myths, or tales of how the earth was formed, such as 'Earth Story' or 'The Triple Mirror'. In Steiner-Waldorf schools, the major festivals of the calendar (Christmas, Springtime, Midsummer or St John's Eve, and Michaelmas) are celebrated with story, drama, movement and music. There are also specific stories with the qualities needed to celebrate each season. Further, teachers can also choose stories, as they do in any school, to reinforce co-operative behaviour, raise awareness of bullying, and address the challenges that can occur in a group of people, including death.

Seventeen Camels

There once was a Bedouin family who lived in the desert. They bred camels and lived in their tent woven from camel and goat hair. There was an old father and three fine sons. One day the father gathered his sons together,

'My dear sons, I am getting old, and it is time to tell you how to divide up my camels between you when I am dead and gone. To my eldest, I will give one half of them; to the next, one third; and to the youngest, a ninth.'

A short while later, the old father died. His sons were all very sad, but the day came when they wanted to share out the camels. The eldest took it upon himself to organise this, so he counted up the camels left by his father. There were seventeen.

'Well, I shall have half of these!' he declared, but his brothers laughed,

'How can you halve seventeen?' they asked.

'What about my third,' the middle son demanded. But the others laughed again, because they realised they could not split seventeen into three.

'What about my ninth?' asked the youngest.

Then they were all puzzled because nine would not go into seventeen either.

'What can our father have meant?' they all thought. And they pondered this problem night after night round the fire in the cool desert air under the stars.

One evening an old man was seen travelling towards them on his camel. As is the custom of hospitality in the desert, they invited the traveller to sit round the fire, and gave him something to eat and drink. The brothers began to tell their visitor about their problem. How were they to divide seventeen camels by a half, a third and a ninth? The old man smiled.

'I will lend you my camel, so you can divide them up, and you can return it to me later.' The brothers looked at each other in disbelief, but next morning they borrowed the old man's camel. Now they had seventeen plus one, which made eighteen.

'Well, that's easy,' said the eldest brother, 'half of eighteen is nine!'

The middle spoke up,

'And one third of eighteen is six.'

'Well', said the youngest, 'one ninth of eighteen is two, and I am happy with them.'

The eldest son then made the reckoning,

'Nine plus six plus two, why that makes seventeen! We have divided up our father's camels, and can return the borrowed one!'

Being boys of the desert, they soon realised why this was, and gave one loud laugh. The old man joined in, until it was time for him to go on his way... with his own camel.

When I first went into schools with stories, the emphasis was on 'speaking and listening'. The reasoning was that listening skills would be developed by hearing compelling stories, which would engage those pupils who tended to misbehave and not concentrate. By re-telling some simple stories, or reporting on stories they had heard, the children would practice speaking. But my experience of the sessions told me there was far more going on than this. Storytellers nationwide colluded in finding any officially approved way to get traditional stories into schools, knowing that they were bringing hidden treasures into a rather dry national curriculum. Since then, I have told stories in schools for 'multicultural education', as I have lived for a short while in both Africa and Asia and can tell stories from traditions there, complete with ethnic clothes and musical instruments. In predominantly white English schools this gave children an opportunity to experience other cultures; in more multicultural schools I sometimes helped pupils reconnect with aspects of their heritage. But stories 'have wings', by which I mean often the same root story can be found in every culture: 'Cinderella' is the most well-known example, as a form of it can be found in most places. Stories can convey culture, but they also exceed their cultural boundaries. I always felt I was taking far more than one prescribed aspect of story with me into schools.

In adult life we continue to need stories to encourage us, and help us meet our challenges in a creative way. We begin our life journey with the energies and optimism of youth, but need guidance and inspiration as we continue through it. In the absence of wise elders at our side, we can turn to the advice of our ancestors recorded in stories, both personal and traditional. Traditional stories are experiencing a revival at present with good reason: they contain instinctive knowledge of the human struggle with free will, and also the eternal moral values that are the basis of all religions. All this is presented inside a mysterious, magical mixture that gives deep satisfaction to both listener and teller. Adult life brings the responsibility for others, with the need to make decisions that will affect future generations. In bewildering modern times, as technology pulls us forward into global communication possibilities, we need to be sure of what we are communicating, and of our words and intentions. Stories can help give us clarity.

Recently, I went to morning yoga class in a Cotswold market village considered to be conservative both in politics and lifestyle, the kind of class that might be held in hundreds of village halls in the UK. In the final meditation the yoga teacher said, 'Drop all interfering thoughts, be here and now in mindfulness.' At the end of the class I went to the wholefood shop in the next village. The shop assistant mentioned that tonight her husband was away, and she knew she would not bother to cook good fresh food, but would probably just have a sandwich. 'I hope you enjoy the rest from cooking,' I remarked. 'Ah,' she sighed, 'I find it hard to relax. I have friends with a mindfulness bell that they ring when they need to drop all other thoughts; I need to get one.' So I received two prompts to be mindful, meaning to drop all worrying idle thought and come home to myself to the present. The prompts were not only for me, but for the other yoga students and the shopkeeper, and out in ever more widely rippling waves of exchange between people. Such conversations would once have been considered 'way out', but today in the 'conservative' Cotswolds, such ideas are alive and thriving! Change is at work all the time, fuelled by the daily conversational stories we tell each other.

Why are stories so special? Stories can creep under locked doors, hide under beds to come out at night into the dreamer's sleep, they can blow around playgrounds bringing showers of smiles, they can be sipped with beer in pubs and carried out, they can be freely taken away in chip shops, they can be medicine in hospitals and amusement in market places. Stories can resound in those who have heard or told a story, and grow like dried yeast put into warm water, lifting the spirits, giving healing and wisdom to whole societies, nations, generations.

Truth and Story

One Saturday morning, Truth woke up, brushed out her long dark hair, pinning it back with hair slides and ribbons, and walked naked out of the house into the town. As she walked up the high street, she saw people she knew. But when they saw her, they gasped, turned their heads away, darted behind doors, disappeared up alleyways and sidled off into shops. The sight of naked Truth made them recoil in fear. By the time she reached the top of the high street, teardrops had welled up in her eyes; she felt rejected.

She pressed her nose onto the steamy window of her favourite café, where inside people were gathered round listening to and laughing with Story. In his colourful coat embroidered with panels of pictures, animals and symbols, he was an attractive and entertaining man. As his story ended, he looked up and noticed naked Truth outside, and saw how beautiful she was, just as the tears began to roll down her cheeks. Story was big-hearted. He got up, opened the door and welcomed Truth in. 'Here, take this cloak and wrap it around yourself, I have plenty more.'

Truth took the beautiful sea-green cloak, embroidered with birds, animals, castles and characters, dried her tears, and came to sit beside Story in the café. Now stories came into her mind, and soon she was telling tales she barely knew before. People drew close; they wanted more, and hours passed as together Truth and Story enthralled their audience. That was the beginning of their romance. They are now happily married, and rarely appear alone.

2. What is a fairy tale?

The folk tale is the primer of the picture language of the soul.

JOSEPH CAMPBELL

Fairy tales are the deepest revelation of the folk mind and feeling.

RUDOLF MEYER

A fairy tale is a hero or heroine's journey on the pathway to sovereignty, often requiring the help of magical animals and guides to overcome challenges. Typically, the hero or heroine has parents or stepparents who are ill-meaning or foolish, necessitating a journey. Because the hero or heroine has a good pure heart, animal guides assist them in overcoming superhuman obstacles, including death, and thus in gaining empowerment through conquest or marriage. A fairy tale contains psychology, sociology and history. The wisdom in fairy tales almost certainly comes from the pre-Christian, pagan and shamanistic past, when most people did not read or write and needed these potent stories to understand events and themselves. They are not cosy pretty stories with fairies in them, or just any story you would find in a child's reader or on a library shelf. They are tales that tellers in the ancient past created and honed to serve the people; listener and teller together wanted – from the depths of their psyches – to hear them. These tales answered a deep longing for understanding and resolution of feelings, and gave wisdom and guidance of a profound kind.

Examples of classic European fairy tales are 'Beauty and the Beast', 'Rumpelstiltskin', 'Rapunzel', 'Cinderella', 'The Goose Girl', 'Iron John', 'The Devil with the Three Golden Hairs', 'The Frog Prince', 'The Juniper Tree', 'The Firebird and the Horse of Power', and there are many, many more to be found in the Brothers Grimm and other classic fairy story books. Russia, Norway, Sweden, the Czech Republic, South America, Africa, Japan, China, Tibet and more countries all have fairy tales passed down through generations of storytellers.

Primal wisdom

Wilhelm Grimm, who, with his brother, contacted and listened to so many old tellers, wrote about:

> ...fragments of belief dating back to most ancient times, in which spiritual things are expressed in a figurative manner... The mythic element resembles small pieces of shattered jewel, which are lying strewn on the ground all overgrown with grass and flowers, and can only be discovered by the most far-seeing eye. Their signification has been lost, but it is still felt. (In Colum, 1983)

What did the old tellers' imaginations tap into when they told these stories? Rudolf Meyer (Meyer, 1988) calls it 'ancestral blood', meaning the intuition before rational thought, which came from the closeness of people and animals in early tribal life. So close did our ancestors live to the very source of life and death all around them in their cooking, spinning, weaving, farming and hunting that they had an unquestioning sense of life forces. They felt the wonder of the higher self and coloured it as the goose girl's golden hair, which she could not hide forever, and as the golden hair of the king's son in 'Iron John', discovered by the observant king's daughter. Golden hair is both royal and the sign of a person on a great journey to hone the higher self or soul. Gold uplifts us; it is rare treasure. The old tellers 'dreamed solutions to the secrets of the world', says Rudolf Meyer. Meyer calls the ancestral wisdom 'dreaming' because it is not rational scientific thought. It is primal wisdom: the early form of what we might now call 'awakening', but without the educated rational mind that we now have.

The old fairy tales were developed before science changed how humans conceived of the world around them. Before the middle ages, for instance, the body of a dead person was too sacred to tamper with, being a vehicle to help send the person back to the spirit world. But, in the early modern era, science in the form of surgery sought to analyse the human physical form, forcing the new medical scientists to steal dead bodies for dissection. Such actions and the understandings that flowed from them constitute a radical shift in thinking. In order to understand the inspiration behind fairy tales, we have to step into the way of being before science by disengaging our logical thinking.

Similar motifs are found in traditional stories from cultures geographically far apart. In the English ballad of 'Tam Lin', the young Tam Lin is under a fairy spell and he gives his lover instructions to break it. At midnight on Halloween she is to drag him from his white horse and hold him in her arms while he changes form into a lizard, a snake, then a red-hot iron (which does not harm her), until he resumes his human shape. It is clear in the story that the fairy queen changes his form to try and keep him under her dominance. Compare this to the Russian tale 'Frog Zaravina', in which a prince shoots an arrow and gains a frog under a fairy spell as his bride. In order to finally break the spell, he must hold her while she changes form from bird, to lizard, to snake, then to an arrow that he must break into three pieces, before she appears in her human form. This transformation must have been recognisable to our ancestors, perhaps as a ritualistic release from 'fairy' or unseen forces.

There are numerous repeated motifs, such as falling into a well to find deeper knowledge, walking through a doorway and being showered with either gold or ashes according to your integrity, rolling a golden ball to find the way, being able to talk to animals, three drops of blood or candle tallow giving power, going to fetch the water of life, wearing a cloak of invisibility, and so on. All this points to widely held ancient beliefs – a religion in picture language – which had consistent ways of depicting what the storyteller wanted to say. The stories would have been understood across Europe and northern Asia and indeed beyond.

Eternal values

Fairy tales have values that transcend the particular time and place of their origin. For example, injuring or killing someone is punished by appropriate injury, banishment or death. Cinderella's bullying step-sisters had their eyes pecked out by birds from the tree at her mother's grave. The malicious king in 'The Luck Child' seals his own fate by imitating the hero's journey but because he takes the oars of the eternal ferryboat man, he fails to return from his trip to find gold. Similarly the self-seeking king in 'The Firebird and the Horse of Power', who sets impossible tasks for the archer on pain of death, does not reappear from the boiling cauldron. The serving maid in 'The Goose Girl', who usurps her mistress to become a royal bride, proclaims her own death sentence when asked by the prince. The mother who chops off the head of her son in 'The Juniper Tree' is crushed by a heavy millstone.

There is a whole category of stories with innocent, guileless protagonists. An unpromising boy, perhaps unskilled, lazy, inexperienced, usually without wealth or status, goes on a journey and succeeds where others fail, because he is honest and kind hearted. In the French story 'Three Golden Apples', the youngest son is not practical but he is honest and trusting, and so, though his older brothers fail, he cures the sick princess with three golden apples. The Russian story 'Vanya' is similar: Vanya shares his food with an old person and he is the one to meet the strange but gifted companions on the way to the king's palace, complete the set tasks and win the princess as his bride. Honesty and kindness win through.

In the 1980s, I used a West African story called 'The Kalabashes of Kouss' in a shadow puppet performance to raise awareness of the famine in Ethiopia and knowledge of Africa in general.

A hare meets a kouss goblin in a field and asks for jewellery for his wife. The young goblin tells the hare to go to his parents' home, but warns him not to mention anything unusual that might happen there, and to be sure to choose the smallest gourd as he leaves. The hare is invited into the goblins' cave, where the old mother goblin plucks a chicken, puts the feathers in the stew pot and throws the chicken on the fire. When she brings in a load of sticks on her head, the sticks pick her up and lay her down on the ground. The hare says nothing, eats the stew and chooses the smallest gourd. When he gets home he finds the gourd is full of jewellery and richly woven cloth. The hyena sees the jewels and tries to follow in the hare's footsteps, but exclaims loudly when he sees the bizarre happenings in the kouss household and chooses the largest gourd. When he gets home, he finds a cudgel in the gourd, which beats him soundly.

I performed this play many times and absorbed its wisdom. The story echoes in my mind when I am in an unusual situation where it is better to accept what is going on rather than question what I do not understand. To learn something new and find treasure, we must first open ourselves to experience new things.

The unexpected or the reverse appears in stories in order to dislodge the rational mind. In North American Lakota culture this process of disruption is found in the antics of the satirical clown Heyoka: you need the chaos of Heyoka if you are too complacent or too fixed in your behaviour or ideas.

Kindness, honesty, respect, unselfishness and a refusal to harm or kill others are the human qualities that will lead us on a path to 'treasure or a royal wedding'. Such values can be found in all religious creeds.

The soul's journey

In the story of 'The Two Brothers', the brothers begin their journey from home together but then must take different paths; they both put their daggers in a tree so that each can see if the other is well by whether the dagger shines or not. They care for each other as brothers, but must obey their unique destiny alone. Perceval, in the grail story, grows up deep in the forest, isolated from society because his mother fears that if he became a knight he would lose his life as his father did. But while out in the forest he sees a group of knights ride by and the sight of them so enchants him that he must leave the security of his home and follow the knights alone. The constant journeying in traditional stories gives reinforcement of what we come to discover about life: we journey alone. Stumbling, foolish, royal or gifted, it is our *own* intuition, passion and determination that takes us through our life.

However, in all the questing and journeying stories, there are helpers. The hero or heroine sets out and meets an old person on the path who tells them how to overcome the challenges they will meet. The hero or heroine may save animals, birds, bees or even trees, which perform for them the superhuman tasks that they must accomplish in order to win sovereignty. Does this resonate with our everyday lives? Are there unseen guides and forces around us, who help and steer us along our unique path?

In many great fairy stories the royal hero or heroine spends some time as a servant in another kingdom before their qualities are recognised. This functions as an initiation test for the royal traveller: if they can be both royal and humble when serving in another land, they will gain an understanding of everyday life and ordinary people, and also a purity of soul. Jesus, Mohammed and the Prince Siddhartha (who became the Buddha) all spent time with ordinary working people in a humble way. Nelson Mandela spent twenty-five years in prison to emerge as the leader who could bring an end to apartheid in South Africa. Gandhi was not a great orator, but spun and wove his own cloth and cultivated his own food as an ordinary person did; this way of living gave him qualities that enabled him to unite the diverse castes of India and lead them into independence. Prophets spend time wandering alone or retreating quietly to perform simple daily tasks, not just for reflection, but to learn what it is to serve others and to become aware of the eternal in the ordinary. Are fairy tales describing part of a spiritual quest? Of the great fairy tales themselves, Rudolf Meyer says,

> the path which leads from compulsion into the freedom of individuality, is hard. It demands the renunciation of all shining wisdom: the soul must go through poverty and the wilderness before it can become a queen. (Meyer, 1988)

We may never be sure of a definitive interpretation for fairy stories, yet we may feel that they are deeply satisfying.

Children do not question the truth of these wonderful stories. They enter into the world of myth with wonder and enthusiasm, and sigh deeply when they feel refreshed by them. I first witnessed this as a puppeteer. The children looked at the puppets, enchanted, and whatever mistakes I made changing hands and props mattered little. Today I use glove puppets without a puppet booth and act out a story on a simple table with the minimum of props. I am aware of young children entering another state of mind when they listen deeply to a story. Children who are about nine years of age will often ask, 'Is that story true?' They are emerging from a child's way of experiencing the world into a more tangible one. I usually reply that it is true in Story World.

> Basically children never doubt the inner truth of what is offered nor the existence of fairy-tale heroes and heroines, as long as the narrator is really united with the truth-content of the fairy tale. (Meyer, 1988)

What is certain is that fairy tales are told to children all over the world and they absorb the fairy-tale motifs in their formative years. These are a literary creation with a massive and fundamental effect on generations of people. As parents, carers and teachers, we naturally want to pass on the stories that had meaning for us, or that we heard from a loving parent – that is a natural impulse. The teller must have some connection to the story to give it the feelings children will relate to. Exact meaning is not so easily communicated. Children themselves will often ask for a particular story that has meaning for them, and careful observation while sharing the story may reveal the reasons.

Two highly influential books which explore the meaning of fairy tales are Rudolf Meyer's *The Wisdom of Fairy Tales* and Bruno Bettelheim's *The Uses of Enchantment*. Each of these writers has their own viewpoint, yet both agree on the importance of fairy tales for the development of children. Meyer applies an anthroposophical analysis, while Bettelheim employs a Freudian and Jungian one. Each has written their particular interpretation of the stories in detail, and I am aware that my writing here adds my own slant to their meaning, with the influence of contemporary ideas and my own experience. Perhaps we have lost from our conscious minds our picture language and the intuitive understanding of these ancient stories, but when we hear them we are still free to let them resonate within our deep psyche. All interpretations illuminate in some way, but my experience is that what gives meaning to stories is our personal *response*.

3. Stories for transformation and healing

> If only there were evil people somewhere insidiously committing evil deeds, and it were necessary only to separate them from the rest of us and destroy them. But the line dividing good and evil runs through the heart of every human being and who is willing to destroy a piece of his own heart?

ALEKSANDR SOLZHENITSYN

In tales, the main character sets out, poor or rich, and sooner or later faces almost insurmountable challenges. This catches our interest. How are we to cope with the seemingly impossible situations facing us? Our heroes and heroines must experience difficult times, parallel to our own, giving us a way to feel their despair, grief, fear or bewilderment, and to turn this into courage, persistence and hope, as well as success in overcoming obstacles. After empathising with a story hero or heroine, our deep psyche is then satisfied that our life can progress. Most of the wonder tales give us these elements and more: 'Vasilisa and Baba Yaga', 'The Firebird', 'Perceval', 'The King of Ireland's Son', 'The Goose Girl', 'The Juniper Tree', and many more. From the ancient Russian stories and Arthurian legends to the Brothers Grimm collection and modern classics, these stories set their hero or heroine impossible challenges.

Some of these fine stories involve killing a helper in order to use their bones as a ladder, then bringing them back to life with special water or by following specific instructions (such a pattern occurs in 'King of Ireland's Son'). Here is the life/death/life element identified by Clarissa Pinkola-Estes in her groundbreaking book

Women who Run with the Wolves. It is an element in which she finds Jungian and feminist insights, regarding it as the strong force that stops our lives becoming stagnant. Our deep psyche knows this, even if we consciously do not want to know it. Our lives are not defined by the secure frame of the embroidered sampler hung on the wall showing, 'Home Sweet Home'; a life is more like a river, constantly fluid, often taking us to places we did not expect to visit. The Indigenous American tradition gives us a view of this life/death/life sequence from a perspective no European could imagine in the story of 'Jumping Mouse' (the complete story is in Chapter 9).

A mouse, a very ordinary creature, whose vision of life is limited, hears the sound of the river of life, which compels him to begin his journey into the terrifying unknown, with the possibility of eagles preying on him should he stray from the familiar cover of trees and bushes. He is offered help only if he gives away one of his eyes – his way of seeing. Only if he trusts to the life/death/life process can he complete his visionary journey. When completely blind, an eagle does swoop down on him, but he then becomes an eagle himself, with the clear sight and lofty view of the finest of birds. The story tells us this is the journey of life: find the river and always be ready to give up your way of seeing.

Now we begin to recognise the psychology contained in ancient stories. Those old tellers knew instinctively, with amazing insight, what their listeners hungered for after days of physical toil and the challenge to survive. It was not practical instructions or new enterprises they needed, but encouragement to face the trials of their deeper selves. This would lighten the physical exhaustion and reassure them that their greater lives were worthwhile. To meet our inner struggles with vision, hope, healing and humour: this is what we crave.

A potent transformation story is 'Angulimala', which tells of the wild brigand who wore a necklace made from the fingers of people he killed, and so got his name: Finger-necklace. He only knew how to kill, until the Buddha showed him that love and compassion were stronger than destruction. Angulimala finally reveals that he was brought up in the lowest caste, the untouchables, with great violence and never knew caring. He becomes one of the clearest and most astute monks in the Buddha's ashram. This is an old story, and it fits the founding claims of modern psychology and therapy. A violent person is someone who needs help; violent and abusive behaviour is a state that the deep psyche wishes to change. Satish Kumar has embroidered this story with compelling detail as *The Buddha and the Terrorist*; it appears more briefly in *Buddhist Tales*.

When I think about some of the stories that have had strong meaning and importance for me, I find that they do not have a pattern or recipe: they are surprising, astonishing and capable of shaking me to my depths. One of these stories tells of Pwyll and Rhiannon from the *Mabinogion*. During the mid 1980s, I made a glove-puppet show of this story and performed it in the ancient castles of Wales; I had a passion for it, which I wanted to play out. Nowadays that story is history to me, and I no longer need to perform it; I have found other quite different stories.

The story tells of the love affair between Pwyll, prince of Dyfed, and Rhiannon, a horse goddess from the Otherworld. Rhiannon wants to marry Pwyll and so avoid having to marry according to her father's choice. But after they finally succeed in being wed, Rhiannon fails to become pregnant. She falls out of favour with Pwyll's counsellors until, after several years, she does give birth to a son. Midwives are sent to attend to her through the night of childbirth but they fall asleep and, upon awakening, find the baby boy has been taken away. Fearing for their own lives if the truth of their neglect comes out, they take a newborn puppy, kill it and say Rhiannon herself killed and ate her own child. Rhiannon is punished by standing at the castle gate every day for the next seven years, telling her story and offering to carry anyone who wishes it on her back through the gate. Fortunately, the child is deposited at a farm nearby by the same clawed hand that took it, and is brought up by the farmer and farmer's wife as their own. The child's likeness to his real father, Pwyll, is recognised as he grows, and he is taken to his mother, who is at last relieved of her punishment.

This story is raw and harsh, and presents events that could not happen in the everyday round. That is the power of it, and why I became so involved with it. It enabled me to say things that could not otherwise be said; it helped me to feel the extremes of sorrow and punishment that Rhiannon went through. I myself went through several years of having miscarriages just before this time, and the story was cathartic in a very positive way. It took me through feelings of guilt and self-blame, while being a historic performance to enliven the ancient castles of Wales. There was also the enjoyment of staging the puppet show, the pleasure of creating props, script and puppets. What remains with me is the astonishing realisation that I was bold enough to choose this story at that time, with only a whisker of realisation of my possible motives, which did not grow into understanding until much later. The ending of the story is that the child is found: all would be well, and I would find a child. In a potent story, there is the experience of raw painful feelings, and also their resolution. It is transformational, although not necessarily in the way that we first imagined. It is certainly therapeutic, with the therapist being our internal guide who chooses the story. I have sought stories that have this potential: though of course I can only speak from my own sense of potency, and each person will sense which are their own transformational stories. What follows are some potentially transformational stories I have found, honed and told.

Maybe, Maybe Not

Once there was a ferryman who rowed people across the river Severn between Arlingham near Gloucester and Newnham on Severn in the Forest of Dean. Like many ferrymen, he was a man of few words, who understood the world that he carried in his small boat.

One day a young mother got into the ferryboat at Arlingham, clutching her sick baby. She said to the ferryman, 'My baby is sick with fever, isn't that terrible?'

The ferryman picked up his oars, and replied, 'Maybe, maybe not.'

While the mother and child were in the Forest of Dean, the Black Death broke out in Gloucester, but the baby avoided close contact with the disease and it survived.

Later, a man got into the ferry at Newnham in a foul temper:

'I have paid all my savings to have my son apprenticed, and what has he done in the first few weeks? Why, he climbed a tree to get apples, and fell out and broke his leg. How will I afford a doctor as well? Isn't that terrible?'

The ferryman merely replied, 'Maybe, maybe not.'

Within a week, the King sent soldiers into every town and village to recruit for the Holy War. Because the man's son had broken his leg, he could not be recruited, and so was spared the destiny of many fine young men.

You yourself got into the boat and told the ferryman about the shocking, painful and terrible things that have happened to you. 'Isn't that terrible?' you ask.

He picks up his oars and replies, 'Maybe, maybe not.'

Is there an unseen advantage underlying what has happened to us? Is a crisis also an opportunity? Of course we have to surrender to what happens to us but, when we realise this, before we burn the map we are navigating by, we may see a good way forward. The 'Maybe, Maybe Not' story can be light-hearted fun, or help someone face difficult times. It is often enough to jog someone out of fearful inertia.

Here are some more short, potentially transformative stories. They are jewels in my story bag, waiting to be pulled out at the right moment.

I heard this story of 'The Prince and the Ring' from a friend, Sheila MacCartney, and I have not come across another source.

The Prince and the Ring

There was once a young prince who was in love with a princess. He went to her father, the King, to ask for her hand in marriage. The King looked at him, and thought he was too young.

'Take this ring and wear it for a year and a day. If you can keep it safely, then you will have proved you can look after my daughter.'

The ring was very large and fitted very loosely round the prince's young fingers. All that year he wore the ring, often clenching his fist to keep it on his finger.

One day, as he walked beside a lake, dreaming of being with the princess, he tripped over a rock, flinging the ring far into the water. Immediately he strode into the lake, straining the mud through his fingers for the lost ring. The water grew muddier and cloudier, until he no longer had any idea where the ring might be. He sat down on the rock, put his head into his hands, and fell into deep despair. How could he marry the princess, now he had lost the ring?

He sat there for quite a while, until the murky water cleared. As he looked up he saw the ring, lying on top of the mud under the water, a little way off. Now he began to think clearly. He slid carefully off the rock, rolling it slowly towards the ring. When it was near enough, he leant over the rock and was able to pick up the ring without clouding the water.

At the end of the year he presented the ring to the King. He married the princess, and there was a great celebration.

When they were finally alone together, the prince told the princess about how he had nearly lost the ring in the lake. She was an attentive princess, and said, 'The rock that tripped you up was the thing that you used to retrieve the ring; what tripped you was the very thing that helped you!'

They lived happily together, and the princess grew into a very wise queen.

A New Dawn

As darkness began to fall, an old, old man made his way towards the forest. His back was hunched, his bones clattered, his joints rattled, but steadfastly he walked on. He knew where he was going. He hobbled into the forest, through the enfolding dark trees, until he came to a light. In the middle of the forest, there was a cottage with a light in the window. He came to the cottage and opened the door. There was a blazing fire in the hearth and, beside it, an old woman in a rocking chair. She beckoned him to her with a welcoming smile. She took him up in her arms – he was all skin and bone – and began to rock him. She sang to him in a low, soothing voice. She sang and rocked him, rocked and sang. As the night drew longer, the man grew younger: now he was a young man, and quite soon his arms were plump and rounded, his legs were chubby and sturdy, his cheeks rosy and full. He had become a young toddler. He no longer had need of the old woman, and pushed himself off her lap to the floor. Just as the pink ribbons of dawn threaded themselves through the dark trees, he toddled to the door, pulled it open and leapt high into the sky.

He became the morning sun, that new day, flooding the land with new light.

This simple story can be embellished with a song as the old woman rocks the man through the night: deep, slow, sonorous healing. I have told it beside a bonfire on New Year's day, so that the old man symbolises the old year. For a more complete experience, the past year could be briefly recounted, to celebrate or transform things that have happened. In my experience, people want to be taken on this journey at important festive times: even at snappy-happy parties, people will draw this story from you and listen with deep, quiet intensity.

The Man Who Was Sad

There was once a man who was always sad. Nothing could please him, he wasn't interested in anything, and so he had no idea what to do with his life. He decided to go and see a holy man. He set out on his journey and passed through a forest where he met a very lean and hungry wolf. The wolf asked him where he was going, and when he heard he was going to a holy man, the wolf asked, 'Will you ask him for me why I am always so hungry and can never get enough to eat?' The man agreed, and walked on through the forest and began climbing the mountain.

On the mountain path was a spindly tree with withered branches, and it called out to the traveller, 'If you are going to the holy man, will you ask him for me why my branches are so withered – why am I not growing tall and strong like the other trees?' The man agreed to do so, and walked on till it got dark, when he realised he wouldn't reach the cave of the holy man that day.

He saw a light ahead, and knocked at the door of a small farmhouse. A young woman opened the door and offered him a bed for the night. During the evening they talked together beside the fire, finding each other very pleasant company. When she heard he was to visit the holy man she asked, 'Will you ask him for me why it is I am so lonely?' Agreeing to do this, he set off early the next morning to the cave of the holy man.

The path was rough and rocky, but the man finally found the cave. He asked the holy man why it was that he was so sad, and couldn't get on with his life. The holy man replied, 'Everything that pleases you is there waiting for you.' The man asked for the wolf, the tree and the young woman, and received answers for them. The man now had hope in his heart, and was impatient to get back to his life to see what was waiting for him. He rushed down the mountainside. As he passed the farmhouse, the young woman was waiting for him:

'Wait, wait, what did the holy man say for me?'

'Oh yes,' replied the man, 'he said if you got married you wouldn't be alone.'

'I would like to get married,' the woman said, 'but up here I don't meet many men. But I like you, would you marry me?'

The man was in a hurry, but replied, 'I like you, too, but I've got to find the things waiting for me in my life; I'll be back when I have time.'

Rushing down the mountain path, he came to the withered tree, which called out to him,

'What did the holy man say for me?'

'Ah, yes,' replied the man, 'your branches wither because there is a treasure chest buried under your roots, blocking them.'

'Please will you dig it out; wouldn't you like to have the treasure?' begged the tree.

'Yes, I would like some treasure, but I haven't got time just now: I have to get back to my life to find what is waiting for me,' replied the man, running on down the mountain and into the forest. There the hungry wolf was waiting:

'What reply have you got for me?' he asked.

'Ah, yes,' said the man, 'he says you should eat everything in front of you.'

And so the wolf did.

This version of the well-known 'Man Down on his Luck' is an Indian one, which I heard from Professor K.N. Dwivedi. I feel this version has an open gentleness about it, which is refreshing.

A well-known story often called 'The Frog Prince' can be found as the very first tale in *Grimm's Complete Fairy Tales*. (Grimm, 1993) It tells of the youngest and most beautiful daughter of a King, who takes her golden ball out into the garden to play with. The ball drops down a deep well, and only the frog who appears at the edge of the well can retrieve it. The princess promises him anything to get her ball back; the frog demands to sit at her table and sleep in her bed with her. She agrees to this in word only, and rushes back to the palace with her ball. But the frog persistently follows her, jumps onto the dining table, and hops up to her bedroom after her. The princess puts him in a corner, but he hops into bed with her. She gets so angry that she throws him at the wall and he is transformed into a handsome and kind prince. He reveals that he was put under a spell by a wicked witch, and only by sharing the princess's food and bed could the enchantment be broken. They get married and ride away in a magnificent carriage driven by his faithful servant, Henry. As they drive to his kingdom, the iron bands round faithful Henry's heart break open with happiness at his master's release.

This story is almost certainly an old tale told to help young women with their first sexual experiences. I find it demonstrates a way to transform aspects of myself I do not like. If I cannot stand taking the 'slimy frog' to my 'bed', then I need to throw it against the wall until it transforms into something I would like to 'take to bed' with me. This transformation might be self-acceptance, changing my habitual behaviour or attitude.

The Tree at the Crossroads

In a wild and desolate place there was a large tree beside a crossroads. It was one of the main routes between two populated areas, and many travellers passed that way. Under the tree lived an old man.

One day a young traveller came from the east of the country and took rest in the shade of the tree. When he saw the old man, he asked him,

'What are the towns like to the west of here?'

The old man asked, 'How have you found the towns you have come from?'

'Well, I did find some work, and the people were friendly enough,' replied the traveller.

'The towns to the west are the same,' replied the old man.

Days later, a traveller came from the west, and seeing the old man, asked,

'What are the towns like to the east?'

'How have you found the towns you have come from?' ventured the old man.

'Well, I didn't find much work, and the people weren't very friendly,' said the second traveller.

'The towns to the east are the same,' replied the wise old man.

The Cracked Pot

At the edge of a village in India, an old man lived a simple life. Every day he would make the journey to the river with his two pots to collect water.

One day when the man had gone out of his hut, the new pot began speaking to the old pot.

'You know, you have got great cracks in your sides, and you leak out half the water our master goes every day to collect. It's time he got rid of you and bought a good new pot, like me! You're just an old crackpot!'

The cracked pot was downcast. When the man returned home, the pot got up enough courage to say to him,

'I am an old, cracked pot and it's time you got rid of me and bought a new one.'

But the old man turned to the cracked pot:

'When I come up from the river, you will notice I always put you on my left shoulder. Then when you leak half your water as I climb back up, you water the seeds I have sown there. Haven't you noticed the beautiful flowers that blossom beside the path? They give me so much joy and inspiration, that they make the journey seem short, and my burden light. I know all the other village people pass that way too, and notice the flowers. So, you see, I never want to change you. You do the watering for us all and are perfect as you are!'

The old pot beamed, and was happy.

The Hollow in the Stone

A young man rushed towards the flooding river. He had tried everything, and nothing in his life seemed to work. His ambitious business plans had failed and his childhood sweetheart had married another man. He felt desperate, and decided he would end it all by jumping into the turbulent part of the river so he would be swept away.

He waded out from the bank to the huge rock against which the main torrent of water rebounded. He stood on the rock, gauging the swell of the water, determined that he would at least make a success of this last task, when a group of women from the nearby village came to fill large earthenware pots. Each woman in turn filled her pot and put it on a flat stone on the riverbank, before arranging a ring of material on her head and balancing the heavy pot on top. The young man kept very still so he would go unnoticed. The women were in any case more interested in chatting with each other.

As the last woman lifted her heavy pot on her head, the sun shone on the stone they had used. He saw that it was not flat but had a hollow in it from constant use.

'Even that hard stone can be shaped by constant use,' he thought. Then other thoughts went through his head about how he could rekindle his business, and how persistence could work for him too.

He got off the rock and went home to try again.

How an African Hunts

A young man wanted to hunt game, so he went to an old hunter and asked him what he should do. The old hunter told him,

'Do not eat breakfast, do not eat supper, then you will catch the animals.'

The young hunter came away thinking,

'The silly old fool, what does that matter, except I won't have any energy to chase them.'

So he ate a good breakfast and took food with him as he set out for the wild forests and savannahs. Days of searching and trailing animals followed, but the young hunter caught nothing. He returned to the old hunter to tell him.

'Have you eaten breakfast? Have you eaten supper?' repeated the old one.

'Well, yes, I have,' confessed the young one.

'Don't eat breakfast, don't eat supper, then you will catch something.'

The young hunter now took this advice as a last resort; he was desperate to succeed. He set out on an empty stomach into the wild, with just his spear. Days went by, as he slept under cover or in trees, hunting by day and night. He was hungry; he became thinner, and more desperate.

Then one early morning, just as he felt he had no more strength left in his body, he saw a gazelle. He followed it through scrub and small trees, aimed his spear, hit it in the chest, and brought it to the ground. He proudly dragged it back to the village, to share with his family and tribe.

He visited the old hunter again to tell him of his success. The old hunter nodded,

'The animals can smell when you are close to death and will sacrifice themselves for you.'

This story was told to me by my Ugandan friend, Sam Mukumba. Undoubtedly, it is a young man's initiation story. But the feelings it evokes in us are relevant to the current 'green revolution', in which we begin to respect and involve ourselves with nature, plants, trees and animals. It is a story that works wonders on teenage boys in an outdoor environment.

The Rabbi's Gift

There was once an old monastery in beautiful wild countryside. But the monks had grown old and the monastery had become dilapidated. Walls were falling down, the garden was overgrown, even the prayers were often forgotten and not said at the correct time. Not many visitors came anymore, and no new postulants came forward.

A Jewish rabbi was visiting the area and decided to call on the monks in the monastery. He was welcomed, and given all the hospitality the frail monks could muster:

a simple supper and bed. The rabbi said very little, but walked around seeing what was happening in the decaying monastery. The next morning he gathered the brethren together, telling them he had something to say. The monks gathered in the chapel, and the rabbi spoke.

'I have just one message for you all: one of you will be the next Messiah.' He then got on his horse and rode away.

One by one the old monks began to wonder who the Messiah might be.

'It must be Brother Francis, he is so kind to everyone; except of late he forgets other brothers' names,' thought one.

'Brother Simon must be the Messiah because he knows everything... He doesn't always listen these days, though,' thought another.

'It's probably Brother Peter,' another pondered. 'He sings like an angel; mind you, of late he gets the verses mixed up, and can no longer read the music.'

Each monk considered each of his brother monks in turn, and then realised it could well be himself!

The brothers began to sweep and clean the monastery in a new way, fit for a new Messiah. They often bowed their heads to each other in anticipation of discovering this new revelation. They made sure prayers were said correctly and evensong sung in tune. Those who were able tended the garden more ardently, planting flowers and vegetables.

One Sunday, a large family came to visit the monastery, and sat in the chapel to hear the service. They noticed that the old place had a fresh atmosphere, that the chants and prayers were beautifully said, and they were moved by the sincerity they now felt. The following week, this family brought their friends, and they too witnessed the calm, peaceful but buoyant mood of the monastery.

Soon the chapel was full of visitors every Sunday, joining in the hymns and prayers. Months passed, and then a young man asked if he could come and join the order. Now other young men wanted to come, and in a short time the old monks found they had young hands and hearts to help them keep the monastery going. Walls were repaired, new songs and prayers were learnt, new recipes were cooked up in the kitchen, until the old place sang again with happiness and harmony.

All this from the rabbi's one gift!

I like this original version of 'The Rabbi's Gift', but it begs to be re-translated to any task that needs a shine. While this story pivots on respecting the divinity within each of us, it represents this as restoring the monastery and monastic life. Energising a place with love does really work. It is easily verified that people will care for a place that looks cared for, while they will allow rubbish and decay to grow in one that is not. Do not read this without trying it out yourself: find a place in your street or front gate or garden where people pass. Perhaps put out the rubbish in a caring, more enticing way: decorate the rubbish or recycling bin, put a new cover on it. Watch and see what happens to your neighbours' bins and others down the street!

The phrase 'Let Nature be your teacher' is from Wordsworth, but the idea is also in Indigenous American philosophies, where it shows in the use of animal and nature guides in stories (for example, in the story of 'Jumping Mouse'). Many fairy stories, such as 'The Frog Prince', also use animals as metaphors.

A swan glides over a lake. Its pure white, feathered wings held like a crown, its neck arched forward as it swims through the water. The perfect image of purity, the essence of the soul. Beneath the water it propels itself with two large, black, webbed feet, strong and active. Dark and light move together, in a dynamic relationship. We want stories to show us how to use those 'dark' thoughts and feelings inside us, transforming them into 'light' ones. This image could be used to make many healing or 'medicine' stories, and here is a simple one I have composed. With this as a beginning, I would embroider the story as needed for a particular person or group, using a creative instinct for what would touch them.

The Girl with Big Feet

There once was and was not a girl who had big feet, enormous feet. She couldn't wear girls' shoes, she had to wear men's shoes: broad, clumpy, heavy men's shoes! How she longed to wear shoes laced to the ankle with straps of leather, and look like Aphrodite. She hated her feet and how the other girls looked at her, teased her, or, at best, politely turned away. So she slouched along, head bent, shoulders rounded, hoping not to be seen by anyone. She wanted to be a worm, living underground in the dark.

One afternoon she wandered out by the estuary. The tide was ebbing, showing tongues of sand each side of the flowing river. There in the sand were big feet marks: bigger feet than her own! Webbed feet, determinedly set into the wet sand. She followed them till they melted into the ebbing water. When she looked up she saw a swan, its neck and head in one gracious curve, its wings held like a crown. The sunlight on its perfect white feathers and the ease with which it glided along enchanted her.

Quite suddenly, three other swans flew out from the trees over the river. The swan on the river began to beat its wings, edging its body above the water. Then she saw its huge black feet, now paddling the water very fast. It rose above the water's surface and gave a great cry as it joined the three flying swans, 'Ayyaaammmm, Ayyaammm, Ayyaamm.'

The girl felt her own feet sinking into the black mud and thought she would drown, but the beating of powerful wings all around her lifted her above the river.

The uplift of air pulled her body till she thought of holding her arms out to steady herself, as if she too had wings. She had become part of the triangular formation of the swans in flight. Something held her naturally in place as they flew over the estuary. She felt warm sunlight on her back and the freedom of air around her as she learnt to move in a new way, nestled between the swans. She stretched out her neck, she balanced herself with her arms, she began to enjoy flying! In formation they swooped, changed direction, yet flew together in exhilaration over the estuary. 'Ayyaamm, Ayyaamm, Ayyyaamm', they called.

Suddenly, a cloud came over the sun and she found herself at the edge of the river, her feet deep in mud. She turned towards firm ground and somehow heaved herself out of the soft mud. The call of the swans echoed again in her mind until she realised what it was saying: 'I am, I am, I am.'

Now she turned and headed home. As she walked, she planned how she would make a white frilled dress, how she would cut and sew it.

It so happened that there was an end-of-year party at school. So the girl bought some material and began making the dress she had carefully planned. Then she thought,

'But, my feet, whatever can I wear on my feet?'

It was her mother who persuaded her not to give up. She said that since it was summer, the girl could have bare feet at the disco and, more than that, she could decorate her feet with rings and bells from the market. The day arrived, and she stood in her new white swan dress, feet washed, scented and decorated. She stood up straight, shoulders proudly holding her head upright. As she walked, she felt the suppleness of her own body as she had felt in the air, and began to move in a new way. At the party, everyone noticed her.

'How graceful she is, she moves just like a swan!'

Since that day, she has spread her swan wings, found her own beauty, and glides along with poise and confidence; perhaps you will see her.

Stories for tranformation for young people come from Susan Perrow, a storyteller and teacher living in Australia. She has created many short healing stories as responses to challenging behaviour. She often uses corresponding animals as metaphors. Her stories have titles such as 'Dishonest Dingo', 'Whingeing Whale', 'Greedy Possom', 'Pesky Pelican', 'Restless Red Pony', and many more. With her experience of children's behaviour, and affinity for letting her imagination run free, she writes simple but effective stories appropriate for each development stage: narrative nature stories for the very young, emerging as animal fables for those beginning school, going into fairy tales for older ones, seven and upward. Rhythm and rhyme come flowing into her creations as rivers of natural healing, and yet she presents this with guidelines that bring the task within most parents' and teachers' capabilities.

4. Teller and listener

The perfection of the present moment is something we touch.

THICH NHAT HANH

If, as a parent, babysitter or friend, you have read or told a bedtime story to a child, you will know the feelings generated by this storytelling. It is an intimate, personal communication like a conversation with a close friend. The child may wish to tell their own tales of what happened during the day, as is natural for us all: this is a very important part of storytelling – giving affirmation to the child. (Mellon, 2000) Then the teller says, 'Once upon a time...', and begins to satisfy the appetite of the young listener. The child's breathing may become deeper and more regular, their eyes softly focussed and body relaxed. This can be observed by any parent, every day. As an adult, check your own feelings and state of mind when hearing a good story. When I listen to an inspired storyteller, the teller 'disappears', as the story itself becomes the vehicle of communication; I melt into the chair, room, even voice of the teller, and enter the world of the story.

My experience as a storyteller over the past fifteen years has been that listeners, children especially, enter another state of mind: a semi-dream state. Their attention is held, a silence falls, they are held by the story, their breathing visibly changes, they seem to 'draw close.' As the teller, I too 'draw close' to them. I notice their response to the story, adjusting the tempo of the story to suit them. Together we adjust to each other, to create a communication space between us. In this space, a new part or ending of a well-known story may appear as I tell it. The audience seems to draw words out of me. If this feeling of response does not happen, I am disappointed, and will try again with a different story. Most storytellers will pride themselves on saying, 'That story just came to mind; that is why I told it.' There are often rational reasons for telling stories, but there may be other intuitive senses at work, nudging the storyteller to choose a particular story.

The extended mind

Rupert Sheldrake is a biologist who has challenged the standard scientific view of the way we see things and the relationship between our mind and brain. In his book, *The Sense of Being Stared At*, he puts very clearly the problems posed by the conventional theory of knowledge and the everyday evidence of our senses which refute it.

> When we see things, where are they? Are they images inside our brains? Or are they outside us, just where they seem to be? The conventional scientific assumption is that they are inside the brain. But this theory may be radically wrong. Our images may be outside us. Vision may involve a two-way process, an inward movement of light and an outward projection of mental images. (Sheldrake, 2003)

Our common sense tells us that what we see is a mental construction: things are really where they seem. This is just the beginning of trusting our senses.

> Our perceptions are mental constructions, involving the interpretive activity of our minds. But while they are images in our minds, at the same time they are outside our bodies. If they are both within the mind and outside the body, then the mind must extend beyond the body. Our minds reach out to touch everything we see.

Sheldrake calls this 'the extended mind'.

> The extended mind may have measurable effects. If our minds reach out and 'touch' what we are looking at, then we may affect what we look at, just by looking at it. If we look at another person, for example, we may affect him or her by doing so.

Sheldrake experiments by getting people to stare at other unwitting subjects and seeing whether those stared at become restless and turn their heads to check behind them. Indeed, we can all try this by staring at the back of a stranger in a shop, train or bus. Sheldrake reports that eighty percent of the people he has asked informally have experienced a sense of being stared at. (Experiments continue, and you can get involved or find out further details online.) Sheldrake discusses how loving looks are acknowledged. In India, many people visit a holy person for a 'darshan', a look that gives a blessing. The 'evil eye' is found in literature, along with phrases like 'if looks could kill', 'she looked daggers at him'. He gives a wonderful example of watching a vixen command her pups with merely a look, and no sound. In my experience as a teacher, it is wise to cultivate a commanding 'look' over the whole class, and 'eye' a misbehaving pupil rather than raising a tired voice. You can recall your own experiences of looking and being 'eyed' by another.

I am interested in Sheldrake's idea that our consciousness extends beyond our body. The communicative power of the storyteller's body language is widely recognised, as is that of an actor or actress, culminating in the superb storytelling skill of a mime artist. Something is expressed and communicated by body movement and facial expression fuelled by the intention of the artist. By 'intention' I mean what the storyteller wishes to communicate, what they 'have in mind' when they tell a story. It covers the feelings invested and overall sense of a story. Mere language without the feelings expressed through the body and mind is like the computer-synthesised messages we are now so familiar with on corporate telephone answering machines. Full expression is given with language, body and mind.

It is not only by looking at others that our minds are extended. In the dark we can sense another's presence: there are party games in which this is played out. Healers can see or feel the aura of a patient as a field of energy around them. Kirlian photography can show the energy fields around a human being. In his book, Sheldrake quotes a tai chi teacher: 'in man's early history our senses would have been far sharper than they are now.' This refers to our awareness of what is going on around us: our 'cat' or 'dog' sense. Have we lost the sharpness of our senses in our 'civilised' society, and can the timeless art of storytelling rekindle it?

I recently told the story of King Midas to teenagers, and found that the ending changed its emphasis. King Midas is given donkey ears by Apollo, for being so foolish as to judge Pan's pipes to be better than Apollo's harp. King Midas hides his ears under a tall hat for a while, but his secret is out when the barber cuts his hair and has to release the burden of keeping this royal secret by whispering it to reeds. These reeds are cut to make flutes, and they sing out his secret. At last Midas has to reveal his donkey ears. I found myself saying, '"You will be the king to listen to our secrets," said a child. King Midas was pleased with this, and so became the Listening King.' The teenagers in the audience quickly reinforced this, and confirmed that they had secrets they wished to tell. I had picked up their need to tell 'secrets' (what they felt about life, adults, their current challenges) and put it into the story. The traditional story does not have this ending.

When a story is told and listened to in a good and beneficial way, as it should be to fulfil its purpose, then teller and listener touch each other's minds, or consciousness. They are in conversation. This is my experience, and it brings great satisfaction to both teller and listener. Young children do not normally fake interest, pleasure or satisfaction, and so telling stories to them can verify the power of connection when stories are told. 'Deep sighs and unusual silence fall on satisfied children,' writes Nancy Mellon. (Mellon, 2000)

If this is so, then the storyteller has a great responsibility to create a clear space in themselves and to have good intention in telling a particular story. I have learnt this from making many mistakes, and returning home from a storytelling session feeling very disconnected, uncomfortable and sometimes in physical pain, until I realised what went wrong with the communication. As a teacher, I know that I must start from where the pupils are, not from where I think they are or should be. As a storyteller, I know that I cannot force a story onto an audience, even if it is one I have just heard and want to try out on my unsuspecting victims! There are adult story circles where new stories can be passionately retold. A story can be healing for me, but others may or may not benefit from this need to tell it. Being clear about a personal interest in a particular story leads to the wise use of it.

Kinesiology of telling stories

Here is a way for storytellers to investigate how their inner state of mind affects not only their own well-being but that of others. It could be a good warm-up for a storytelling group. You will need a group of people interested in storytelling. The participants need a short simple story they are prepared to tell. Ask three participants to come out of the room, away from the rest, and give each of them a storytelling intention to hold in their minds as strongly as they can. Then they re-enter the room, and each tells their short story (possibly the same story) keeping in mind the intention they have individually been given. Afterwards, the audience in the room can give their reaction to the three tellings, and try to guess what the intentions behind the thoughts were.

Here are three thoughts/intentions:
1. Listen to my story and the way I tell it with all the metaphors and creative words I use.
2. Come into my enchanting world of story and be bewitched.
3. I wonder what words this group of people need to hear?

Follow up this exercise with a discussion of the power of intention while telling a story.

There are many variations to this. Imagine different types of audience, and how they would affect the stories chosen and the way they are told; for example, an audience that is very elderly, or bereaved, or homeless, or shocked and traumatised, or a wedding party, and so on.

The Listener

There was once a famous violinist who played in all the prestigious concert halls in great cities around the world: London, New York, Sydney, Paris, Amsterdam, and more. At every concert, sitting somewhere in the front row, was an old man who loved the violinist's music so much that he followed him everywhere. The violinist noticed him, although after a performance he was always surrounded by fans and admirers, so he did not meet this one faithful follower.

One evening, the violinist prepared to play, putting rosin on his bow and tuning the sonorous violin. He walked onto the concert platform, bowed to his audience and began to play. Somehow the notes did not resound as best they could, and at the end of the first piece the violinist became unsettled. He looked along the front row for his usual tireless follower, but saw just one empty seat. Bowing and apologising to his audience, he quickly left the stage, lifted his priceless violin up in the air and brought it down with force against a steel bar, smashing it beyond repair.

That one old man had listened to him so deeply that now he was no longer there, the virtuoso violinist could not play his best.

5. Storytelling skills

The universe is made of stories, not atoms.

MURIEL RUKEYSER

Everyone is a storyteller; we tell each other stories every day. But if you have a feeling for the rhythm and rhyme of words, a passion for traditional stories and a desire to communicate, then you may develop the skills to become a storyteller to whom people turn for wise, witty and satisfying words. There is a great difference between *reading* a story and *telling* a story. When reading, the words are fixed by being written on a page; in contrast, telling a story is open to improvisation from the imagination so that the teller can adapt the tale to the audience, entering the teller–listener connection (as discussed in Chapter 4). This has great implications for communication, healing and spiritual development.

What are the steps a storyteller needs to go through? Here are some stages of story skills: choosing a story, story bones and story craft.

Choosing a story

A story must grab your interest. I remember going to a good library, where books were displayed in various areas. In the children's section, a large book caught my eye. It had rainbows on its cover and an African look about it. Its title was *Mbaba Mwana Waresa;* it was a Zulu myth story about the rain goddess. It delighted me.

I had no particular use for it, no group of children or adults to tell it to, but I knew I had to learn it. As it was on display, I couldn't borrow it, so I read it several times and took notes on it, especially the African names. Over the following days, I said the names over to myself. While washing up, I told the story to myself. I got out musical instruments to make rain sounds to make it more enchanting. I looked in reference books to check for any other sources of the story and aspects of the rain goddess. Then, ready or not, I tried it out on a friend, corrected anything I had forgotten or mistaken, and told it again: three times is the recognised number of times to tell a story before it becomes 'yours' and you take the responsibility of being a carrier of that story. Since then, I have told it many times to children and adults, in schools, village halls and yurts. It has grown with me, and changes and evolves the more I tell it.

This is a good start to telling a story: being drawn to it, feeling passionately about it or having an urgent compulsion to re-tell it. You may be looking for a story for a particular purpose, and have to take one up quickly, or you may find yourself in a situation where you have to make up a good story on the spot. These are all very good starting points.

There are some powerful and enchanting short stories. Start small and grow into the longer, more complex folk tales, myths and legends. You may be lucky enough to hear a story being told at some of the festivals, or in the Highlands and Islands. The Society for Storytelling in the UK is now well established, and there are monthly storytelling circles in most towns and cities at which you can both hear and tell stories: check their website for the diary.

There are now several websites that are helpful in finding or researching a story (see the 'Useful Websites' section at the end of this book).

Chapter 7 (Ages and stages) discusses choosing an age-appropriate story.

Story bones

Stories are usually remembered in pictures in the mind. From this, words flow to describe the picture. So each time you tell a story you will use different words, and each person uses different words when telling the same story. Sometimes there are difficult names to learn and remember, but most storytelling is describing a picture or scene, largely improvising the exact words as you tell. This is the key difference between reading and telling a story, and it has profound implications, which I discuss later.

Taking a story down to its basic narrative enables a beginner to remember it more easily, and a more advanced storyteller to fill it out in various textures and colours for different audiences. One way into a story is to read it several times, put it away, and then think it through in its simplest form: its bones. The bones can be written down, but if you are going to tell the story very soon after reading it, it is better just to record the story in pictures in your mind, and then re-tell it using your own words. Doing this opens up the imagination much better than writing it down, and it develops your memory very quickly!

Story bones can be remembered as connected to the fingers of your hand: place the thumb onto the first finger and imagine the first scene, then touch the thumb to the second finger while thinking of the next scene, and so on. When you want to tell the story, touch the thumb to the first finger to recall the first scene, then thumb to second finger for the next scene, and so on.

Here is a good short tale taken to its bones. It may not be suitable for the group you are concerned with; I present these exercises to illuminate the process of telling stories and to consider the storytelling qualities needed for different age groups.

The Three Golden Eggs

Bare bones

A poor Burmese woodcutter dreams of a tree fairy smiling at him, finds and cares for the tree, and receives a gift of three gold eggs.

He loses one to a magpie, one to a fish and the third is stolen by a neighbour.

Next day he retrieves one egg from the magpie's nest, his son catches the fish, and the neighbour is shamed into returning the stolen egg.

He and his family are now well off, but he continues to thank and care for the tree.

Story bones

A poor Burmese woodcutter lives with his wife, son and daughter.

He dreams of a tree fairy smiling at him, finds the tree, cares for and talks to it.

A nest appears in the tree with three golden eggs in it.

Overjoyed, he thanks the tree and walks, looking at the eggs.

A magpie flies off with one.

When he bends down to drink from a river, the second gold egg rolls into the water and is swallowed by a large fish.

The third gold egg he gives to his wife, who puts it in the large rice jar in the backyard.

A neighbour sees this and steals the egg away during the night.

Next day, the woodcutter climbs a tree to get fruit, and retrieves his first gold egg from a magpie's nest.

As he returns home, his son shows him a large fish he has
  caught.
Cutting it open, they find the second gold egg.
The neighbour hears their joy, and returns the stolen third
  egg to the rice jar.
They now have enough money, but the woodcutter thanks
  and cares for the tree for the rest of his life.

Fleshing out the bones

Exercise 1

Tell this story to young teenagers about twelve to thirteen years
old. Make sure you give it a credibility that will engage teenagers,
and a pace to keep their interest. If you know your audience well,
introduce it in a way that connects them to it: 'What do you
think the Himalayas are like? Would you like to go there? What
do people do there?' Teenagers are interested in what is real in the
world, as well as needing to recognise and exercise their emotions –
a need stories and drama can meet (see Chapter 7).

There was once a poor woodcutter who lived beside the
forest in the mountains of Burma, at the foothills of the
Himalayas. He had a wife and son and daughter to support,
with only the income from selling wood. Like any rural
folk, the family had chickens, a cow and goat and a small
patch of land for a garden. But the woodcutter was anxious
to earn enough money to send his children to school and
college in the big town some distance away: that would cost
him much more than he made at the moment. With all this
on his mind, he went to sleep one night and dreamt that a
beautiful fairy was smiling at him from a hole in a tree.

Next morning he walked into the forest with his saw
and axe, and looked for the tree. When he found it, he

took off dead branches, swept around its roots, and began speaking to it. Every day he passed the tree, and told it how much he admired it, leaving a small present for it.

One morning, he sat under the tree, with his back to its trunk, gazed at the dawn light shining through the branches swaying in the breeze, and told the tree all that was on his worried mind. Some time passed, as the woodcutter listened to the tree's reply, said in the way a tree can speak to a human – perhaps not in words at all. As he got up to go, he noticed a nest in the branches. Inside were three golden eggs! He picked them up, thanking the tree, and walked along the forest path dazzled by gold. He had never seen so much gold in his life before! Why, there was one egg for his daughter, one for his son – that would see them through college. The third one he and his wife could keep for their old age.

As he walked on, daydreaming, a flash of black-and-white feathers snatched one of his eggs and flew off with it.

'My golden egg! How foolish I am, I have already lost one!' he said, as he put the two remaining eggs into his pockets and continued on.

He had been cutting wood for some hours when he felt thirsty, and knelt down beside a river to drink. As he bent down, one of the eggs rolled out of his pocket, down the river bank, into the water, and was swallowed whole by a large fish.

'Give me back my golden egg!' he screamed at the fish, but it had already swum swiftly away.

As he went home, he felt the one remaining golden egg in his pocket. 'I'll give it to my wife for safekeeping,' he decided. He told his wife all the adventures of the day, and gave her the remaining egg. She took it to the backyard, lifted the lid of the large rice storage jar and buried it deep in the rice grains. As she handled the egg, the evening sun shone onto it, sending a flashing shaft of gold into the eyes of her neighbour, who was feeding his chickens nearby.

When all were asleep that night, the neighbour crept into the backyard, lifted the lid of the rice jar, found the gold egg, and stole it away. Next morning, the woodcutter's wife went to the rice jar to get rice, but could not find the egg she had hidden there the previous evening.

The woodcutter's heart was heavy as he realised he had lost every one of the eggs given to him by the tree. He picked up his saw and axe, determined to work twice as hard that day, to try and make up his loss in some small measure. As he passed his favourite tree, he apologised for losing all of the eggs it had so generously given him.

The woodcutter did work hard that day. Becoming hungry, he climbed a large mango tree, stuffing his pockets with juicy ripe mangos. He came up to a large nest made of twigs, and saw a gold egg nestled among the magpie's eggs.

'That's my gold egg the thieving magpie stole yesterday,' he said to himself, as he picked up the gold egg and put it deep into his pocket.

He turned to go home and, as he reached his house, his son rushed out to meet him.

'Dad, dad, look at this large fish I caught today; we'll all eat well tonight!'

'Sharpen the knife, and we'll cut it open and clean it before we cook it,' said the woodcutter.

They lay the fish on the kitchen table, and began cutting it open. Out of its belly rolled a gold egg.

'That's my second gold egg I lost yesterday!' said the woodcutter.

They barbecued the fish with garlic and chillies, and invited all their neighbours to the feast. Everyone ate well and enjoyed themselves, singing, dancing and telling stories way into the night. The thieving neighbour was there too, and went home feeling very ashamed for taking something from his generous host. When all were asleep, he stole back into the yard, and returned the gold egg to the rice jar.

Next morning, the woodcutter's wife lifted the rice jar lid, dipped her gourd ladle into the rice and brought up a gold egg. The woodcutter could hardly believe his eyes: a large smile lit up his face, and has hardly left it to this day.

He gave one egg to his son, one to his daughter, and the third he and his wife kept for themselves. But he continued to visit his favourite tree in the forest to thank and care for it.

If it be true, if it be not true, take some with you and bring some back to me.

Exercise 2

Re-tell this story to children under eight years old. Include rhythm, repetition and pace. Find and dramatise the high points of the story. Bring it to a satisfying conclusion.

There was once a woodcutter who lived with his wife, son and daughter at the edge of the forest. He loved the trees and always asked permission from each tree he cut down.

One night he had a dream that a tree fairy was smiling and waving to him from a hole in a tree. Next day, he searched for the tree he had seen in his dream, and when he found it he gave it a small gift, told it how lovely it was and tidied up the space round its roots. Every day he was in the forest, he gave the tree something and spoke to it. The tree fairy, who indeed lived in the tree, grew fond of the woodcutter.

One day he was worried, so he sat under a tree with long cool leaves, saying, 'Tree, tree, listen to me.' A breeze blew through the branches,

'I'm listening, I'm listening,' it seemed to say.

'I am so worried. How will I send my children to school – I don't earn enough money. How will my family manage if I am ill?'

'Look in my branches, look in my branches,' said the breeze.

The woodcutter got to his feet, and on the lowest branches he saw a nest, and in it three golden eggs. He thanked the tree as he picked up the eggs. Never had he seen so much gold, and as he walked on he was dazzled by the sun shining on the golden eggs.

Suddenly there was a flash of black-and-white feathers, and a magpie flew away with one of the eggs.

'My egg, my egg, come back with my egg!' cried the woodcutter.

He carefully put the other two eggs into his pockets. Off he went to work with his saw and axe. He felt thirsty, so he went to the river, knelt down on the bank to drink, when one of the eggs rolled out of his pocket, into the water and was swallowed up by a large fish.

'My egg, my egg, come back with my egg!' cried the woodcutter.

He turned back homewards, to give the third egg to his wife to keep safely. When he got home, his wife took the last golden egg and put it in the large rice jar in the backyard, safely replacing the lid on top.

But their neighbour had seen the flash of gold, just as the egg was hidden in the rice jar. That night, the neighbour crept into the yard, lifted the rice jar lid, and took out the egg. The next day, the woodcutter's wife went to take out some rice to cook for their lunch packs, but she could not find the egg.

Now the woodcutter was determined to work hard. He set off with his saw and axe, until he came to his favourite tree. 'Yesterday, you gave me three golden eggs, and I have been so foolish as to loose them all.' The tree sighed in the breeze.

As he worked in the forest, he saw a large mango tree heavy with juicy ripe mangoes. He climbed the tree, picking the fruit and stuffing them into his pockets. He saw a large birds nest, roughly made with sticks. It was a magpie's nest. What do you think was lying in the middle? In the middle of the magpie's own eggs was his golden egg!

'That's my golden egg!' he cried and put it deep in his pocket. He hurried home to show his wife, when his son came rushing out to meet him.

'Dad, dad, I've caught a large fish. We will eat well tonight!'

'Put it on the kitchen table and bring me the large, sharp knife,' replied the woodcutter. He picked up the knife and began to cut open the fish. What do you think they found in the belly of the fish? Out rolled the second golden egg.

They were all so happy that they decided to barbecue the fish and invite all their neighbours to come. Everyone ate the delicious fish and rice, and had a wonderful time. They sang songs and told stories until the sun went down.

The neighbour who had stolen the third golden egg felt very ashamed, so when everyone had gone to sleep, he crept back to the yard, lifted the lid of the rice jar and placed the egg on top of the rice. Next morning, the woodcutter's wife came to get rice as usual, and saw the egg sitting on top of the rice.

Now they had all three golden eggs: the woodcutter gave one to his son, one to his daughter, and kept one for he and his wife. They were never poor again. But, forever after, the woodcutter thanked the tree for the gift he had been given.

If my story is true, you can catch its tale!

Story craft

From the examples above and your own storytelling, consider the following aspects in breathing life into a story from its bones.

Pace and dramatic shape

There are no recipes set in stone. The story must come from you; it must be something you enjoy and are comfortable with. However, the pace of the story must meet the energy of the audience. When telling these stories, there are points when words will flow rapidly and dramatically, giving them pace and dramatic shape. For me, this is likely to happen when the woodcutter first finds the golden eggs, and retrieves them from the magpie's nest and the belly of the fish. Experiment with your own re-telling. If there are dramatic and fast-moving times in the story, then there must be quiet and slow times, too. There is sadness when the woodcutter realises he has lost all three eggs, and passes his special tree: this can be a slow-paced time, giving a springboard to when he regains the eggs. Listen to other storytellers and recordings, and note with a critical ear the pace and dramatic shape of their tellings.

Rhythm, rhyme, repetition

Young children like simple and active stories with repeated elements: they are still learning language, and want to hear joyful rhythm, rhyme and repetition. In the second version of the story I have kept the story alive and repetitive by getting the characters in the story to speak. I feel very comfortable with this method, partly because I was a puppeteer before I was a storyteller. Experiment using your own abilities and inspiration. Children appreciate rhyme: it gives them the fun inherent in speech and is essential for language learning. Some stories lend themselves to rhymes. I sometimes 'take a story for a walk' – telling it to myself as I step along – hoping a rhyme will develop.

Remember and re-visit the classic stories you were told as a child, to see how rhythm, rhyme and repetition made them enchanting: 'Three Billy Goats Gruff', 'Jack and the Beanstalk', 'Goldilocks and the Three Bears', 'The Three Little Pigs', 'Rumplestiltskin', and so on. In these classic stories, the repetition builds up pace and suspense before the final outcome. Repeating a story element three times has been with us since we can remember and before. Maybe it represents beginning, middle and end, or maybe it's the rhythm of a complete four-part breathing, with the outcome as the fourth part. (Melon, 2000) Its time-honoured beat works for us all.

Adapting to the audience

Teenagers need strongly told stories with action and pace that keeps up the excitement; they need more realistic details that will engage them in their task of relating to the world. Teenagers have a great need to verify their feelings (see Chapter 7). Young children need repetition and rhyme for the development of their health, understanding and language. For intimate stories, such as bedtime stories, a natural silence needs to fall into which the story can flow. (Mellon, 2000)

Adult audiences are more difficult to classify. There may be something specific about the group that will indicate the source, substance, texture or style of the stories they need to be told. But whatever the specificities of the audience may be, expect the unexpected! I always have two or more stories ready to meet unforeseen needs or circumstances.

Some tellers begin with a short funny story to gauge the mood of their audience. I often ask to be on the door, so I can gain a preview of my audience, and get my intuition and antennae working.

On those occasions when I feel I have 'failed' to engage the audience, there is plenty of good dynamic compost for new growth. Being prepared to learn, and to take the risk of failure is essential: the energy created by telling a story fuels the imagination, so that new ways can be found to re-tell it, days or even weeks after the event.

Being true to the story

In re-telling the story of 'The Three Golden Eggs' in two different ways, I have also kept true to the story bones. I have adapted it to two quite different audiences. I would expect the live tellings to vary again from these written versions, and hope to find ways to give the story still more enchantment, or discover new details and depths in it.

It is said that after telling a story three times, you are the carrier of that story, and have the responsibility of passing it on. There are myths and ancient legends that have content that must be included. These stories feel untrue if such parts are changed. Most Greek myths and Indigenous American 'medicine' (teaching) stories have content and even structure that I would not want to change. A story needs to be respected, and there is only so much that can be changed without creating a distinctly new story, inspired by the original. Indeed, 'The Three Golden Eggs' has content and structure that define the story itself.

Respecting the story

First Nation (North American Indian) tellers advise us to be respectful when we repeat their stories. Their stories have a special place in their culture, which has experienced suppression and decimation by the invasion of Europeans. Many stories are considered sacred, imparting knowledge only intended for specific audiences, and only told at certain seasons or occasions. Many stories have only been released by the elders within the past decade, so that they can be written down.

I have been very moved and educated by some of these stories, and have asked the First Nation tellers I have met how I could tell them, as I wanted others to feel their depth, wit and inspiration. I was told to honour the stories in the native tradition by giving offerings of tobacco or chocolate to Great Spirit. Adapting this to our European way of prayer, I give thanks to the old tellers of these stories before I tell them, so that my intention and gratitude is in my thoughts before I tell it. Because I am familiar with some First Nation customs, I also do ceremonies outdoors with tobacco and chocolate when I can.

Make sure gratitude and the clear intention of respecting the roots and meaning of a story are in your mind before you tell it.

Body language
When you know a story well enough, and have perhaps tried telling it in a story circle, to the plants in your garden, or to your friends, then it is time to bring it to an unknown audience. Now is the time to trust your memory, and create a space in which the audience can respond. Being silent in any way that suits you will enable you to begin this. I sometimes do Chi Kung and Tai Chi exercises. Some way of going within yourself to clear out unwanted doubts and anxieties is what is required. Using an acting technique, imagine your feet growing roots, then you will want to straighten up the spine, focus on your feet and extend energy down beneath them. You will find your voice becomes better seated in your body, and the story seems to come from a more solid foundation within yourself.

Now you are ready to embody the story. Express the emotions of the characters and try and gain an overall sense of the feelings and intention of the story. This will change the more you tell the story, so to begin with you may not have a specific idea of what the story 'means'. Sit with the uncertainty, and allow your imagination and the response of the audience to reveal the depths of the story; there is not just one interpretation to any story. A mime artist tells a story without words. It is not necessary to overload a story with metaphors and descriptions; some stories ask to be told in a straightforward way because their content is so profound, amusing or especially significant. Experiment with gesture, the feelings you put into it, body language and breathing.

I often invite a newcomer to tell a story at summer camp when there is a session for children every evening. One evening a woman wanted to tell the story of Gelert, the dog who was killed by his own master, Prince Llewelyn, who thought mistakenly that his dog had killed his baby son. The story gives the name to the Welsh village Beddgelert, Gelert's grave. It was the one story she was confident to tell. Wishing to encourage new storytellers, I agreed to let her tell it, pointing out that the audience were small children from four years upward, and so she should tell it in a suitable way and not go into gory details over how Gelert died. But when it came to Llewelyn drawing his sword, she graphically described the sword stiking through his neck and coming out the other side. She was evidently proud of her ability to tell it like that. The children froze, and afterwards talked about their pet dogs and how they loved them!

This kind of reality does not belong in stories for young children. They would have accepted a simple unloaded description, 'Llewelyn drew his sword and killed the dog.' Sparseness of this kind leaves listeners free to absorb the greater meaning of that story. Feelings and gestures have to come from the internal meaning of the story, rather than making it into a drama.

You are working towards being deeply connected to your audience. Practice being open-hearted so you offer a welcoming space to your audience. This is not as easy as it sounds, as pre-telling nerves and the adrenalin needed to stand before an unknown audience will be active. I overcome this by connecting to my audience in a small way first. I have experimented with playing the harp, introducing myself, or singing a join-in song or greeting. I use one of these as I feel suits the situation. The harp has a very special sound that opens people's hearts. In truth, I rarely travel without it! It can open closed doors.

Command a silence

Before the story begins, the audience needs to be silent, and it is the storyteller who can bring this about. Using the silence within, bring a silence to the listeners. This sounds daunting, but once tried, you will find that your audience want silence, just as young children want boundaries on their behaviour, and quietness imposed from outside themselves. I try and 'breathe' into my feet, open a space in my chest and heart, imagine a string holds up my head from its crown: this is a yoga technique that makes a clear channel down the spine. The people in the room will feel your connection and opening and hopefully will enter the silent listening space.

The journey of the story does not end there. Each time you tell a story, let the energy of it bring new insights and imagination to refresh the next re-telling: let yourself be a channel for the story.

Beginnings and endings

To mark the entrance into story world, the storyteller can use a nonsense phrase that lets the listeners know they are moving from outer reality to inner reality. Nonsense shakes the rational mind to help release it, so the story can be accepted.

> 'If it is true, if it is not true, take some with you and bring some back to me.'
> 'Long, long ago, perhaps it was yesterday, there was...'
> 'Once there was and there was not...'

The end of a story needs to wake the listeners back into outer reality.

> 'And how do I know this is true? I was there and I heard it myself.'
> 'If you don't believe me, you can go there yourself.'
> 'And you might see them today.'

Listen to how other tellers end their stories. Sometimes the Brothers Grimm have recorded individual beginnings and endings to their stories.

Story aids

Stories for children can have some colourful aids. A story bag, apron, cloak or carpet with pockets in it, filled with stuffed animals, puppets and objects offers lots of participation, and ensures you get immediate interest. Invite the children to take an object and then tell a relevant story. If you have some puppets, these could be played with later, echoing the stories. If you have craft skills, it is great fun to make a story garment, and it focuses your imagination on particular stories in a wonderful way. Using story aids is especially helpful when you begin storytelling, as you are supported by the colourful and stimulating puppets and objects, making you less likely to go unexpectedly blank.

Story workshops for children and adults

After hearing a number of good stories, teenagers and adults will want to become storytellers themselves. Here are some games to stimulate the imagination, loosen the tongue and create a trusting feeling within a group.

Gobble-de-gook

Make up your own language noises. A good warm-up or preparation for this is asking participants to mumble their own made-up language to themselves as they all walk around the room. Once they have discovered their own language and become a little confident in it, perhaps get them to moan to release anxieties, as animals groan for example. This is a recognised way of relaxing and, due to the absence of words, the moaning does not carry weight, but is playful fun. Then they can try greeting each other with their own particular salutations ('Happy Birthday!', 'How are you?', 'Have you heard the news?', and so on) and exchange information, meeting the eyes of another as they walk around the room. Depending on the skills of the group, some pairs could be heard by going into the centre of the circle formed by the group; this often inspires hesitant or shy people. Drama sketches can come out of this if the members of the group are inspired while doing this exercise – let pairs improvise their own scenarios.

Names

Tell a story about your name, its origin, what it means, or anything unusual or amusing about it. Such stories are often interesting and revealing, just as our surnames were ways to distinguish our forefathers' craft (Smith, Tailor, Butcher, etc.). Repeat this for your house, street, town, and more. Use the content to lead people into areas of interest: if someone tells a strong story involving their grandparents, then use this as a group focus and task.

Real stories

'The day I missed/got on the wrong train/bus...' Complete the story. Amazingly, everyone has a funny story to tell, which happened to them, or a member of their family. Some have become family folklore, they are so good!

At present a series of gatherings called 'True Stories Told Live' has become popular. People tell a true story for about ten minutes. Try to find where it is going on near you. There is a lot to learn from this in language, content and personal styles; it also builds community in just one evening.

Lying contest

Construct believable lies about others or yourself and tell them to the group. The listeners vote whether they think it is true or not. Intersperse this with a true story so that the challenge is sustained. Extend this into making up the most unbelievable fantasies served up seriously, with a deadpan face.

Chosen objects

Use objects chosen from a basket as a starting point: say what they are used for, give them a name. The objects might belong within a particular theme, such as wood, stones and leaves from nature;

different hats and gloves; tools of a trade; buttons, threads and material scraps; doctors' or dentists' instruments.

Story in a circle

In a circle of people, each is given a card with a word on it. Each person round the circle makes a story that includes their word. The words chosen depend on the group. Perhaps begin with fairy story archetypes, then give out blank cards so each person writes a word, which they pass to another.

All these games are starting points, and hopefully will lead to quite individual tasks and subjects relevant to the participants: let what comes out of these interactions inspire you to create your own games.

6. Personal stories

There is no one you cannot love, once you have heard their story.

SOURCE UNKNOWN

In our contemporary society there is a greater flow and exchange between people who do not know each other very well, and do not have recognisable roots in common, than in the past. Business demands that many of us speak to others across the country, across the world. Our modern multicultural communications are stimulating, exciting and challenging. But the human heart and soul needs more than this: it seeks to deepen some close relationships. In large, otherwise impersonal organisations, team building is used to improve relationships, and so oil the whole operating wheels of that enterprise. Sharing personal stories is one method of building community.

For older people and those near death, it becomes imperative to tell their personal story. People nearing the end of their life often want to begin writing down their life story, but are daunted by the task. If they have no previous writing skills, they will need help. Note that therapist Damian Gardner advises some caution with people who have had painful lives. (Dwivedi, 1997)

The following simple seven-step method for telling a life story is a good place to begin. I first experienced this method with the storyteller and therapist Kelvin Hall. It can be employed with a minimum of two life storytellers, and a maximum of a roomful.

Seven-step life story exercise

Warm-up

Ask each person to give themselves a fairytale-inspired name, relating it to one significant event in their lives (e.g. Jim Swift Foot, Ben Big Bear, Sylvia Sly Fox etc.). I gave myself the name *Josie Molly Dolly* after a rubber doll I had when young, which was very important to me, and went with me through many adventures. If there is a group of people, get each person to share their name and the reason behind it.

You can also use some of the warm-up games suggested in Chapter 5. This is usually very enjoyable and relaxes a group of participants.

Fairy tale archetypes

Elicit some well-known fairy tales from the group. Point out that extraordinary events and people can appear using magical powers, animal helpers can bring great gifts. Identify typical fairy tale archetypes (the list below gives some examples).

PLACES
  castles
  caves
  fairy rings
  dark woods
  bogland
  lakes
  mountains
  magical gardens
  wells

HELPERS
  magical old people
  talking animals/birds/trees

MAGIC OBJECTS
    swords
    wands
    crystals
    bags
    coins
    potions
    water of life

SEVEN INCIDENTS
Ask people to choose one notable incident from each of these phases of life:
    earliest memory
    early childhood (up to about seven years)
    adolescence
    young adult
    present time
    the worst moment
    the best moment
(For elderly people there could be more phases and steps: adult, middle age, mature.)

Telling the story
Speaking in the third person, each teller begins to link up their seven (or more) events into a brief life story. Working in pairs of listener and teller, the teller begins, 'Once there was a small boy/ girl who...' Their telling must be suitably timed, so that they do not expand on their story too much. For large numbers, groups of four is good, with each getting their turn, and hearing three other life stories. This in itself has a very opening effect on people, as each person realises they are heard. It loosens telling abilities, and leads them to the next stage. Ensure everyone has told their own story and heard at least one.

Re-telling the story

One of the listeners now re-tells a story back to its teller *as a fairy tale*, using all their imagination to enlarge it, and employing fairytale archetypes. Those re-telling need to really get into the mood of greatly exaggerating everything, in a light-hearted way: they need to be given permission to include animal helpers, castles, magic, extraordinary people and events, but keep the solid root and sense of the story heard. The re-telling might start, 'A fine baby boy was born to the King and Queen, and he was well loved and cared for, until his third birthday when...'

Reclaiming the life myth

The original teller then reclaims their life story in fairy-tale form, adjusting anything that they consider is incorrect, and embracing what has illuminated their personal story. They can then tell it as their personal myth, always in the third person. The sharing of another's imagination is very stimulating and usually enlightening, bringing fresh insight into the personal story in unexpected ways. The listener now re-tells their life myth, adjusting anything they feel is incorrect.

Completion

Once the participants have adjusted and accepted their life myth, they can complete the experience by writing, drawing or modelling. This could be a large or small task, depending on their needs. It might just be making a wax or clay model to symbolise the story, or it might be assembling a scrapbook including photos and drawings.

The following story is based on one I witnessed in a personal storytelling session.

Hatching the Golden Egg

A king and queen had a wonderful daughter, but they were so busy tending to their large castle that she spent a lot of time alone. One day she wandered into the henhouse, which was warm with the clucking hens. After that, she would go every day, sometimes speaking to the hens and sitting in their cosy nests of hay. Then it happened that as she got up from sitting in a nest she saw there was a beautiful golden egg in it! She had laid a golden egg! The princess took it to her bedroom and took great care of it.

The young princess grew up and was soon married to a young man her parents very much approved of. He had land and wealth and wanted a wife capable of helping him manage his estate. Married life was content enough and in time the princess, now queen of her own palace, gave birth to three fine children. The young queen was very occupied with bringing up her children and helping with the business of the estate. The children grew to an age where they no longer demanded so much of her time, choosing to spend it with their own friends.

One day, as the queen sat in her closet, she heard a tapping noise. She searched the palace for the source of this insistent sound. As she searched in the depths of a forgotten cupboard, she found the golden egg she had carefully saved since a child. The tapping sound was coming from inside the egg. The queen felt strange new feelings moving through her: sadness at forgetting her golden egg and the loss of her childhood days, then excitement as she realised the egg wanted to hatch! When she told her husband, the king, he scoffed at such an idea, telling her not to be so foolish as to believe a golden egg could hatch.

The queen knew with a certainty beyond reason that the egg did want to hatch: it was of utmost importance to her own well-being. So she crept away from the palace one night with some simple belongings and the egg. She walked through the woods until she came to a forester's hut, which was empty. There she decided to stay. Weeks and months went by, with the egg still tapping.

One moonlit evening, a hole appeared in its shell and a few moments later a golden bird hatched from the broken pieces. The bird began to sing; it sang just for her! Each song was full of longing, sung with haunting melodies. The queen picked up pen and paper and began to write. Poems, songs, plays, novels poured from her pen, till her heart was eased in its fullness.

When she felt ready she returned to visit her husband and children, but she is still writing to this day!

Most people discover that they have many life myths; there are so many aspects to a life story. So the seven-step life story exercise can be repeated.

A community-building exercise I have experienced asked each person, 'What events brought you here?' It was a condensed way to introduce each person: it requires some personal details but also limits them by asking a specific question. The limitations of questions like this, and of the seven steps, give a framework in which people feel secure enough to express themselves.

For elderly people, guidance will be needed to write their life story in a suitable way. Damian Gardner has written an informative chapter 'New Perspectives: Stories and life stories with older adults' in the book *The Therapeutic Uses of Stories*. (Dwivedi, 1997) He cautions against a simple formula for this story work, and gives examples of a sensitive, listening approach. There are many people who do not want to re-live the pain of the past. Using the third person when telling an autobiography may diminish this intensity, but some people may need the experience of a professionally trained therapist to work through their life stories.

My experience is that people have hidden depths of fairy lore and images to use in re-telling a personal story as a myth. If not, help is at hand in Nancy Mellon's book *Storytelling and the Art of the Imagination*. She lists storyscapes, seasons, moods, characters, clothing for power and protection, and more, in this book buzzing with the ways and means to create new stories.

7. Ages and stages: stories in education

Have courage for the truth
With the power of the imagination
And responsibility of soul.

ADAPTED FROM RUDOLPH STEINER'S
MEDITATION FOR TEACHERS

A true educationalist is concerned with helping
self-realisation, for every individual self is a new
message from a divine world. The respect for the
unfolding human 'I' is the foundation of true
educational work and must be given with love, so
that the self can learn to make its imprint on the
tough material of daily life.

BERNARD LIEVEGOOD

I have come across only one system of education which puts
stories at its heart, which considers the phases of development of
the child and gives a philosophy of education to nourish and to
educate for freedom: Steiner-Waldorf education with its roots in
anthroposophy (see Chapter 1).

What is the development of children through school years?
What stories can benefit them at the various stages of their growing
up? School structures give us rough developmental stages: pre-
school, infants, juniors, secondary. Children grow in their bodies,
socially, mentally and emotionally. But there is something else each

parent and good teacher craves: children need experiences that help them 'grow into themselves' – help them to discover and develop what abilities and talents they have, with the passion that will motivate them beyond school. Like plants, from orchids to wild flowers, each individual child needs to grow and blossom. The full development of a human will hopefully always be a mystery, so we will retain our respect and awe of life itself. If we care to be aware of it, there is daily evidence that we are continually developing from birth to death.

Stories have been used for education long before it became formalised in schools; they are the oldest form of education. Some early stories remain in native cultures, such as Maori, Australian Aboriginal, Indigenous American, First Nation, Mongol, Bedouin and many others. Stories from these cultures can be wonderful anchors to contemporary ones, and have their place in the stages of development.

The curriculum in a Steiner-Waldorf school integrates physical, mental and creative activities in a careful and meaningful way. For instance, when the children begin fractions in mathematics, in handwork they do cross-stitching that requires them to count and copy their own patterns. Cross-stitch requires focusing very precisely at the point of the needle, which is a focus needed to deal with fractions. The reflecting of a pattern from one quarter of a sampler to another also develops an inner capacity for careful counting and an awareness of symmetry. Steiner-Waldorf-educated children would accompany work on fractions and cross-stitch with symmetrical physical movement exercises to complete the trilogy of thinking, feeling and willing. Given this level of integration, it is very difficult to separate stories meaningfully from the curriculum as a whole. But for the sake of making this approach to education, with stories at its heart, more accessible to a wider group of people, I offer a tentative guide for ages and stages of development. Steiner himself did give a curriculum for stories through the school years (seven to sixteen years old) and these form the basis for the guidelines below. (see Stockmeyer, 1991)

There is a great difference between reading and telling a story, which Steiner emphasises. For young children beginning school, a story made up by the teacher will communicate in a deeper way, stimulate the child to use language and awaken an interest in reading and writing. It is now standard and regular advice to parents that they should share simple picture books with their children, talking about the pictures in their own way, as appropriate to their child, and enjoying the time together. This is essential if children are to show an interest in reading and writing at school. Parents are a child's first teachers, and have the opportunity to know them better than anyone else.

There is an anthroposophical educational principle at the heart of choosing which stories to tell to children. This is that children develop as humankind has developed: children pass through the stages of social evolution as they grow. If this principle is followed, children acquire ancient wisdom and skills in a meaningful way, passing through the various cultural stages until modern times. This passage takes children up to the alive, creative point of our present-day consciousness; they are then meaningfully equipped to co-create the next phase of evolution. In Steiner-Waldorf schools, stories are also used in other ways, for example, to help children with social behaviour, affirm the changing seasons and to inspire any new project or activity.

Before most people were able to read and write, a community's elders told stories to educate. Just a hundred years ago in the UK there were many who had never learnt to read and write, and there are thousands more now across the developing world who struggle for opportunities to learn these basic skills. What are the ancient pre-literate stories, and why are they more potent than the profusion of modern children's stories that are in bookshops and libraries? Australian Aboriginal creation stories, Indigenous American stories and those from other early communities handed down in oral traditions give us a precious glimpse into the mind of early humanity. Norse myths have given us the days of the week from Tuesday to Friday. Greek and Roman myths give us Saturday,

Sunday and Monday. The brothers Grimm lovingly and accurately collected stories that were still told orally in Germany over a century ago. They deepened their understanding as they recorded them live from the old tellers, who had heard them from older tellers, until they realised that what they heard were the 'scattered jewels' of ancient wisdom told in picture form. The old 'pagan' religion, and an even older affinity with animals, shines through the stories as evidence of early ways in which humans have gathered wisdom (see Chapter 2).

Modern tellers must take the scattered jewels of traditional stories and offer them to the next generation, knowing that much inside the stories comes from a mysterious source. Recognising that a story is never a finished picture, even when it seems neatly framed, is a step towards letting in the mysterious forces which guide storytelling. With this in mind, all tellers stand on the shoulders of past storytellers, yet have the potential to tell a new and powerful story. The tales of Hans Andersen, Padraic Colum and Oscar Wilde also contain enchanting strong images and messages that make them worthy of inclusion in the classical story fountain.

In our global modern world, storytellers can tell diverse stories to make a diverse audience feel included, especially in schools. Telling stories from other traditions can also broaden the horizons of your audience. If you have encountered stories from other cultures, you will have found that they often seem familiar. The Cinderella story is well known for appearing in almost every culture, for example it has similar elements to the Russian 'Vasilisa the Wise,' where Vasilisa is sent by her stepsisters to get fire from Baba Yaga, and the African 'Blue Fish,' where the stepmother starves her stepdaughter who goes to the river for help and finds a bountiful blue fish. There are good reasons to explore beyond Grimms' classic tales.

Early years: three to six year olds

Children are growing physically, developing their arms and legs and their use of language. They need rhythmic and repetitive songs and stories that encourage them to join in, to strengthen their developing limbs, hearts and lungs. Rhymes will help them recognise sounds and experience the fun and joy of language. Simple stories about everyday things and events are just what young ones need.

I remember my father, who was a chef, telling me stories of a mouse who hid inside a large cheese in the larder, while the cat looked for it everywhere. He told it with wit and with his passion for food, and that communicated directly to me. He shared his feelings and love of kitchens with me. He often made bread buns for thirty people, while an ample tom cat sat under the large kitchen table waiting for scraps in front of a great AGA oven: his stories are steeped for me in all these early impressions. When I cook now as an adult, these warm impressions return to me. Those early events, and their surroundings were my first experiences of relating to the world.

If you allow yourself to be with young children, you will find them the best of teachers. Their joy, intense interest with an open face and eyes, will guide you to what they love and what will help them grow. This is a tender responsibility, as children up to the age of about seven are imitators, responding for the first time to the world immediately around them, and laying these experiences as foundation stones on which to build the rest of their learning.

What stories would you tell to these willing but stumbling ones, as they discover and explore their surroundings, and develop their bodies? Familiar classic stories with rhythm and repetition are: 'The Three Billy Goats Gruff', 'Goldilocks and the Three Bears', 'Red Riding Hood', 'The Three Little Pigs', and so on. Recounting the day to a young child, perhaps using the child's name, will affirm them; in their early development, children do not see themselves as separate from everything around them. Steiner kindergarten follows the rhythm of the seasons, to affirm what the children's bodies tell them: that winter is a resting time, spring a budding time, summer an outdoors active time, and autumn a harvest time. There are many creative ways to celebrate the seasons with children, using songs, stories and food. (see Carey and Large, 1982)

Early years children need repetition to reinforce their growing bodies, minds and spirits. Repeating a story at least three times over consecutive days is good practice; more may be appropriate. Children at this age love to act out a favourite story, so telling it and letting them use simple props to act it out and play with it comes naturally to them. They will do this acting out at some stage after hearing a story that touched them, whether formally recognised or not. Giving permission for acting and playing with a story verifies and gives authority to their imaginations. It is this foundation to a child's whole being that will form their creativity. Creativity is in great demand, but building its foundation is often not understood.

Juniors: seven to eleven year olds

The children past early years have gained language skills, and have developed a love for their surroundings and hopefully a sense of wonder at nature's great yearly pageant. They now need fairy tales to 'guide their souls', as Rudolf Meyer says in *The Wisdom of Fairy Tales*. In Europe this will be the classical tales recorded by the Brothers Grimm: 'Snow White', 'Cinderella', 'Beauty and the Beast', 'Jack and the Beanstalk', 'Rapunzel', 'Rumpelstiltskin', and so on. 'The King of Ireland's Son' by Padraic Colum is very popular, as it has all the classic elements of a good fairy tale. A thoughtful and refreshing source of fairy tales is *Quests and Spells* by Judy Sierra. In the multicultural classroom the stories could be world classics: 'Sita and Rama', 'The Birth of Ganesh (Ganesha)', 'The Prince and the Flying Carpet', 'The Living Kuan Yin', and so on.

In their second year as juniors, children are growing more into themselves, preparing for the next phase, but still find a strong connection to animals. The stories recommended in the Steiner curriculum are animal fables, nature stories and fables of saints who had animal helpers. St. Bride, St. Columba, St. Francis and St. Michael are the subjects of stories where animals are helpers. As a girl, Bride walks through an arch and a bird leads her to meet the baby Jesus; Columba walks into the sea at midnight to meditate and the otters come to dry him as he walks out. Siegwart Knijpenga's *Stories of the Saints* tells such stories so they are of interest to this age group. In Steiner's integrated curriculum, children are taken to see animals at a farm, and they then model them in clay. When they are in the older junior years, they will sew small felt animals and stuff them with wool they have seen being sheared from the sheep. Aesops fables are right for this age, and can be expanded from their concise and rather dry form in the Penguin Classics; you may be lucky enough to find a second-hand story book of a fable which has been retold well for this age. I feel a lot more could be done with these wise and humourous tales.

Nine-year-old rubicon

At about nine years of age, children go through a transition from imitating adults and the world around them, to finding their own way to be in the world. They are becoming self-conscious, in the next step to becoming uniquely themselves. They are still very dependent on their family and need the security of a nourishing and accepting home and school life, but the forces within them now demand more self-expression. They become opinionated, frustratingly perverse, changing from a charming child into a more sullen one. They may ask their unsuspecting parents, 'Am I adopted? Are you really my mother and father?' They want and need stories of death and overcoming fear: 'Death in a Nutshell', 'Godfather Death', 'Jack Who Was Scared of the Dark', Baba Yaga stories, *Beowolf.* The stories recommended in the Steiner curriculum are those in the Old Testament: David and Goliath, Jacob and Joseph, Noah's Arc. Nine-year-old children want 'real' stories and these are some of oldest historical ones in both Christianity and Islam. Creation myths can be told, to help children connect to the beginnings of life. These can be found in Australian Aboriginal and Indigenous American mythologies; the best known is probably the Aboriginal story 'The Rainbow Serpent'. There are some good modern re-tellings of the Big Bang, such as: *Earth Story* by Eric Maddern, and *The Triple Mirror* by Chrispeels and Colebrook. Local, real stories are pertinent, because the children of this age awaken to their surroundings. Stories about whatever went on or goes on in the geographical area: farming, fishing, boat building, steel manufacture, coal mining, and building fine churches and houses.

The next era of mythology for people living in the north is Norse mythology. Children and adults are often surprised how the days of the week from Tuesday to Friday refer to Norse stories of Tyr, Odin, Thor and Freya. They are dramatic and fierce stories to tell. The fantastic classic story of Gilgamesh can be enjoyed by older juniors. Then follows stories from Indian, Persian, Egyptian and Greek mythology. These sources are rich and fruitful. There are many collections of Greek myths for juniors, and I have used *Greek Myths* by Geraldine McCaughrean, as it presents the most popular stories in a digestible way, such as 'Persephone and the Pomegranate Seeds', 'The Wooden Horse', 'Theseus and the Minotaur', 'King Midas', 'The Twelve Labours of Hercules', and more. The clearly written books by Roger Lancelyn Green give juniors accessible readers in *Tales of the Greek Heroes* and *Tales of Ancient Egypt*; they also provide teachers and storytellers with these classic stories in a quickly digestible form, in preparation for telling them. In practice, these mythologies can only be touched on, to make children aware of their potential, so that they may follow them up later in their school years.

The story heritage from India is vast and deep; adults and storytellers in the West stumble about in these stories, trying to make them appropriate to children of this age. It is said that our European story heritage leads back to Indian mythology. Most common in schools are simple re-tellings of 'Sita and Rama', 'Ganesha', 'The Buddha', and folktales gleaned from various sources. With the changes in the population of the UK over the past decades, stories from a broad range of cultures need to be told in British schools. Children need to hear storytellers from diverse backgrounds interpreting their ancient heritage. It's important that ongoing efforts are made to support storytellers from diverse backgrounds, and I look forward to reading and hearing their voices.

I have told Persian and Egyptian riddle stories: it is just this challenge and charm of language that is needed for ten and eleven year olds. The usual format is a young girl outwitting sultans, wealthy owners of restaurants, land or animals. *The Wise Little Girl* (Carter, 1991) is a typical example; Angela Carter references it as from a Russian source, but the style is also Iranian and Egyptian. Idries Shah in *World Tales* explains the migration of stories, and gives a riddle story, 'The Riddles', from Turkestan, where Russian and Iranian ethnic groups meet, and 'The Maiden Wiser than the Tsar' from Serbia. There are also many Anglo-Saxon riddles that describe familiar things: an egg, a shield, a plough, the wind, a three-legged stool and so on. A useful book on rhymes, riddles, games and using stories actively, covering the early years and junior range, is *Looking Forward* by Molly von Heider. *Riddle Me This* by Hugh Lupton is a wonderful collection of riddles and more.

In the English language, Greek mythology is thickly woven into contemporary language and behaviour. Pick up an English dictionary to find the roots of common words: telephone, television, psychology, megalith and microscope, tragedy and comedy. The golden touch of King Midas is found in a bank account, goddess Echo gives her name to reflected sound, Heracles has given us Herculean strength, Pandora's box has shown us hope lies under all devastation, and Aesop's fables give us metaphors we use every day without noticing.

Tweens: eleven to fourteen year olds

Teachers and parents all know that children at this age will go through a challenging change from willing student to difficult, argumentative, moody teenager. It is an inner revolution in which the child seeks to find their unique self and express it. Whereas a lively child was interested in reading widely before, now they want drama, to write a diary of their feelings, and be listened to and recognised. They can become storytellers themselves, and so be engaged with story expressively. The earlier foundation of fairy stories is now relied on by the deep psyche, to be used in the teenager's unique way. Whatever way story is used from now on, the older child will want to express their own view on it, and make it their own. This need can be met by creating and dramatising stories.

The Roman civilisation is covered next in the Steiner syllabus. Answering the need of this transitional age group for real events, a study of the Romans can become living history, as there is so much evidence of Roman occupation in the British Isles, from Hadrian's Wall to Bath Spa. Using real places and objects as a starting point, there is a dynamic opportunity for creative drama and storytelling initiated by the students themselves.

Within the developing self-responsibility of the pubescent child is the memory of authority and the need to look up to someone, to have heroes and heroines. The lives of prominent people meet this need: Florence Nightingale, Ghandi, Martin Luther King, Mother Teresa, great discoverers from Columbus to Edmund Hilary, and pioneers of science such as Galileo, James Watt, Hertz and Faraday. The pupils will meet Pythagoras in mathematics lessons now, and Archimedes, Watt and Newton in physics lessons. I still have a copy of *Great Men of Science*, which I read during these years because science attracted my interest. Looking back, I see I was amazed by the creative free-thinking of these men of physics and chemistry; today I use creative free-thinking in storytelling!

These are the years of pin-up heroes and heroines, when pictures from magazines decorate the child's bedroom wall with movie stars, football heroes, pop stars and Olympic champions. This is part of the shaking up of the supremacy of parents and the search for the young teenager's own individuality, together with the discovery of their own sexuality. Parents know that the best way past this phase is through it, by riding the whims of self-discovery of their ever-changing pre-teenager. Most will find their own reading material and will be occupied in writing their own copious diaries.

Echoing the turbulence within is the study of the Middle Ages, the Renaissance and the Reformation. *The Knights of the Round Table* Arthurian legends, and also the mysterious Welsh legends in *The Mabinogion*, could all be presented to tempt the wiles of this age group.

Teenagers: fourteen to eighteen year olds

Parents and teachers will verify that teenagers demand to be treated as young adults by being accorded respect. They must be listened to and heard, and given a place where they matter. They need to have some say in things. What else can adults expect of young people growing into the society they find themselves in? This is a healthy response to growing up.

The Steiner-Waldorf school curriculum reflects this change in status: teenagers are taught world history, what it is to be a world citizen, the origins of myth and drama, economic history, the history of the Middle Ages, and the story of Perceval from the Arthurian legends. The story of Perceval is given to sixteen year olds, as it mirrors their search for a path in life. The young hero unwittingly makes mistakes and often appears foolish in the eyes of others when he goes on his quest. Steiner regarded this story as containing the secrets of the modern initiation path. It is a key story in European heritage and has a wide application to the great plot of the hero or heroine's journey.

Teenagers need plenty of opportunity to discover and express their feelings: drama, discussions, debating, making diaries, painting and music. This is a time when all the stories they have been told as children are bearing fruit, giving them an inner storehouse of emotional flexibility and strength. Now they can begin to exercise their emerging feelings about growing up through being creative. *They* can become the storyteller now.

More challenging is leaving school and taking a place in the world, either with more study, apprenticeship or work. In 1984, I had the opportunity to wander round East Africa for a month on my return from teaching abroad. There, teenage boys are sent out to shepherd the animals, often spending days and nights in wild pasture. They must learn to look after themselves, as well as the cattle, goats and sheep. Young teenage boys were very hard at work selling home-made snacks to the travellers on the Tanzam railway, which at that time went just once a week from Dar es Salaam to Lusaka in Zambia. That journey was the best introduction to Africa I could have had: it was there sitting in the same carriage with me. I was later to meet some boys in a forest near Kilimanjaro, who 'interviewed' me in English, told me which path to go on, and then climbed back up the tall trees they had been foraging in with their pangas under their arms. Their presence, confidence, energy and ease of communication utterly impressed me. Long afterwards I felt like a pale cringing white tourist. Youthful energy harnessed, focussed, appreciated, needed by their communities: this is how the African youths I met were initiated into society. How does it compare with ours? With three-quarters of the prison system currently occupied by people under twenty-five, it is time our society changed its punitive ways of responding to growing up, and created more relevant, productive ones.

I have told stories in the libraries of secondary schools, and sometimes find myself challenged by boisterous teenagers. On one occasion I needed a very strong story to gain the attention of some teenage boys who heckled me. I will always remember the look on a young boy's face when I told this story of finding and keeping your own heart and soul; it was just what he wanted to hear. It is a good initiation story, just right for this age group.

The Black Prince

Once in ancient Egypt there was a very lazy, ugly boy who lived with his mother in a simple hut beside the river Nile. He would laze around all day playing a flute he had made from reeds, or fall asleep on the banks of the river. His mother said, 'My son will come to nothing, he will probably fall into the river and drown.'

One day the boy roamed the streets of the city and came to a high wall he had never noticed before. He was curious about what was on the other side, so he climbed up and sat on the top. He saw that the wall enclosed a very beautiful garden with cool trees, flowerbeds, green grass and a fountain cascading into a pool. Beside the pool there was a young woman, about his age, gazing deeply into the water. He was so caught by the atmosphere of the garden that he began to play his flute. Of course he hadn't learnt any tunes or taken any lessons, so he played just what he felt. He played all afternoon, until it was time to return home. The next afternoon, he climbed the wall again, to smell the scent of the garden, gaze at the young woman and play his flute; he was sure the young woman didn't notice him.

One night he dreamt that he was seated on the wall, playing his flute, when the young woman came over and invited him into the garden. He jumped down to join her and they spent the evening together beside the water. He was falling in love.

One evening, as he returned home, he stopped to drink at a well and heard some old women talking about his special garden. It became clear to him that this was none other than the sultan's palace garden, and the girl he had fallen in love with was Princess Thadmos, the sultan's only daughter.

He knew that a princess could not love a poor, lazy, ugly boy like him, and a cold feeling fell over his heart. He wandered aimlessly through the darkening streets, not wanting to go home, till he found himself by the great eastern gate of the city. This was the gate to which the merchants came, as they journied from the desert. He found a group of them squatting beside a small fire, drinking sweet mint tea, and swapping the stories that travelling merchants tell. It was easy to join them in the descending nightfall. He listened to their talk and something caught his attention: tales of a magician called Habi, who could change people into anything they wished to be.

'Can he change a man's soul?' asked the boy.

'Why, yes, Habi can do anything!' replied one of the merchants.

'But where can I find him?' the boy pleaded.

'Ah, you must go eastwards, out into the desert by the trade route for two days, then find the small oasis with a grove of acacia trees: that's where Habi lives,' came the reply.

The boy stood up, went to the water fountain and filled his water container. It was night-time and cool, and a good hour to begin a walk into the desert. Sleeping by day in any shade he could find, and walking by night eastwards, he came to the oasis of acacia trees. He saw a dingy mud hut and beside it an old, old man with a toothless smile.

'Are you Habi the magician?'

'That is my name,' came the reply.

'Can you change a man's soul?' asked the boy.

'Go to the water and wash yourself, rest a while and then we shall drink some tea together,' came the reply.

Washed and rested, the boy returned to the magician's hut.

'Can you change me into a warrior, a prince who is

fierce and fearless in battle?' asked the boy.

'That I can do,' Habi replied, 'but once changed, I can never change you back.'

'That's what I want!'

'Very well, what have you to give me in return?'

The only possession the boy had was the flute he had made himself.

'I have this flute,' he took the flute from his belt and put it into the old gnarled hands of the magician.

When the boy did not return home, his mother grieved, 'My son has fallen into the river and drowned, so be it.'

She held a simple funeral service.

Time went by, and a year later a warrior dressed in black strode out of the desert. He had such a presence that anyone meeting him was held by his intensity; he was charismatic and undoubtedly a ruthless, fierce fighter.

It so happened that the sultan and his army were camped in the desert to defend their territory. The sultan had lost half his land in a short time, and his army was now small. The soldiers brought the strange new warrior to meet the sultan. He said his name was the Black Prince. The sultan took him into his Bedouin tent where they spoke together for many hours. The prince offered to train the sultan's army and win back his land; the sultan said if he succeeded he would grant him wealth, position and land – whatever he wanted.

Over the next months, the Black Prince took the soldiers through demanding routines, and discussed strategies with their leaders. In six months, the small army won back all the lands of the sultan and more. The Black Prince ordered that any prisoners have their right hands cut off so they could not fight again.

The sultan was impressed. He invited the Prince to come to his palace in one month's time to ask for his reward: whatever he wanted would be his.

Stories of the Black Prince sped before him, and at the end of one month the women of the city decorated the streets with palm leaves and frangipani flowers and crowded every street, rooftop and window from the east gate to the palace. Out of the desert he came, walking slowly with head held high, eyes fixed straight ahead. Every pair of eyes was upon him as he walked towards the palace.

He was ushered into the sultan's court, where the sultan sat on his throne, and beside him sat Princess Thadmos.

'You have served your sultan and your country well, and you may ask for anything you wish as your reward,' invited the sultan.

The Black Prince paused, and a hush fell over the crowded room.

'I wish for neither land nor wealth, but I come to ask for the Princess Thadmos's hand in marriage.'

The princess stirred and stood up.

'Father, if it is your will, then I will marry him, but first listen to my story. There was once a boy who came to the palace garden wall. Every afternoon he would play his flute, he played with so much feeling, it was as if he played all of my feelings too. He was so handsome, like the changing seasons. I used to dream that he would jump down into the garden and we would be together. Then one day he no longer came, and I learnt from my handmaidens he had drowned in the river. Father, I know I can never love as deeply again.'

The Black Prince's eyes looked straight into hers, as he replied, 'I once had a love as deep as yours; I would never force you to marry me.' Then he turned, walked out of the palace, back down the way he had come, and out into the desert, and was never seen or heard of again.

8. Adults: the ongoing journey

When I was in my twenties and early thirties, I thought, along with most of my peers, that people over forty had reached somewhere: 'maturity', or a peak of development, where they had 'arrived'. But when I got to forty and beyond, I found myself in unknown and surprising territory. I had reached a certain maturity, but the goal posts seemed to have moved, and there was yet much further to go. This awoke me to the fact of ongoing, lifelong human development. Because we have choice in our adult lives, and the forces that have shaped each of us are so unique, this development has a wide variety of expressions and it may be difficult to discern the fine threads weaving through all our lives.

The hero's journey

The classic story from Brothers Grimm called 'Iron Hans' has been used by Robert Bly to reunite modern man with his wild self. Bly calls the hero of the story 'Iron John'.

Iron John is a wild man who devours anyone who enters his forest lake, until a hunter drains the pool and discovers him. The king locks the wild man in a cage, but his eight-year-old son lets his golden ball fall into the cage. The prince finds the key and opens the cage door. The wild man carries the boy back to the forest.

The wild man gives the young boy a challenge, to sit beside a well of pure water, yet not to disturb it. Each day he fails, and on the third day his whole head of hair falls into the water, and turns to shining gold. The wild man tells the prince that he must go out into the world and experience poverty. But since he has a good heart, he can ask the wild man for anything, whenever he is in trouble.

The young boy finds work as the gardener's boy at a king's palace in another kingdom. When war befalls the king, the gardener's boy goes to Iron John and asks for an army. He is granted ironclad soldiers and a fine horse, and with these he wins the war for the king, remaining anonymous.

Meanwhile, the king's daughter often notices the golden shining hair of the gardener's boy, and tries to take his cap off to see it. The princess herself asks her father, the king, to arrange a three-day feast for young men to catch her golden apples. The gardener's boy goes to ask Iron John for help, and receives a chestnut horse and red armour the first day, a white horse on the second, and a black one on the third. Each day he catches the golden apple, but does not show himself.

Finally the king sends his men and they capture the boy, and all is revealed. The king asks him what reward he would like, and he asks for the princess as his wife.

At the wedding, a wonderful and wealthy lord arrives: it is Iron John, released from his enchantment.

This is a wonderful old fairy story, which calls up the power of the wild man. It contains the ancient motif of three horses, red, white and black, also found in 'Vasilisa the Wise', and a golden ball, which is in many stories including 'The Frog Prince' and 'The Frog Tzarevina'.

Bly is a therapist and leader of men's groups, and has written a compelling account of using the story for healing the detachment of the male psyche from the powerful, raw wild man instinct. He goes into great detail illuminating many aspects of the son-father-mother relationship that need healing. Bly reports that modern man has 'father hunger': in more traditional times, a father and son would have worked together, maybe just tolerating each other, but the young man would have received 'father food'.

The younger body learns at what frequency the masculine body vibrates. It begins to grasp the song that adult male cells sing, and how the charming, elegant, lonely, courageous, half-shamed male molecules dance.

That is the medicine of being with the wild man. The narrative is very like a male version of 'The Goose Girl'. The hero has to undergo hardship and work as a servant in another kingdom before his gifts can be used and his royalty uncovered. The story itself is so compelling that just telling it to young men, without analysis, at the right time and place, could be very empowering.

'Perceval' or 'Parsifal' is a central story in the Arthurian legends. It is an archetypal story of the journey of humanity: both an outer quest for the Holy Grail and an inner journey in search of wholeness. Perceval is a naïve young man who has been sheltered by his mother and brought up in a forest. With his mother's unwise advice, he sets out on his errand to become a knight in King Arthur's court. After many adventures, stumbling across beautiful women and true love, making many mistakes, becoming lost and surrendering to the unknown path, but developing courage, clarity and tenacity, he is able to ask the correct question of the wounded Fisher King, and so heal him and the surrounding land.

John Matthews, healer, Celtic scholar and shaman, uses 'Perceval' in *Healing the Wounded King*. This book contains a re-telling of 'Perceval' in very clear, usable form, together with healing meditations. Beautifully written, Matthews reveals a shamanic and transforming power within the grail story, where whatever happens to us, we are assured we can finally enter the 'courts of joy'. When the wounded king is healed, the land simultaneously comes back into fullness. Therapist and storyteller Kelvin Hall has also rewritten this story in a clear, refreshing style in *Beyond the Forest*. This book makes the ancient story accessible in the modern world, so teenagers and adults can easily read and grasp it.

The beauty of this story can be felt as it is told or read. It defies exact analysis, as it contains many archetypical images: it can mean different things at various stages of a person's life. It is often used in biography work. Although it is a story of knighthood, and of a quest for honour and purpose, women can also identify with the hero, Perceval. I have heard women say it is a story of experiencing the love we all have within us, given while Perceval dwells in the grail castle; and yet also a reminder of the need for integrity, because we are shown by the hero's struggles that our lives cannot be all joy and light.

The plot of the hero's journey has been traced through mythology by Joseph Campbell in *The Hero with a Thousand Faces*. Literary and extensive though this investigation is, Campbell begins with a story: the timeless, transforming story of 'The Frog Prince'. He offers very clear stages and challenges on the path of initiation, ending with the divine male–female marriage. He maps out in mythology the way we imagine, dream and think.

All these heroic stories and their analyses are wonderful invitations to explore our own journey. Many people feel healed and transformed by these fine hero stories on hearing them, using them as a stimulus in art therapy, re-telling them in their own way in groups, or using them in other ways.

There may be special places that enhance the healing power of a particular story. The place of telling is the choice of the storyteller and the participants. Stories can be told in caves, ancient burial mounds, springs, wells and sacred sites. It is well known that the initiation of young men is effective when the initiate is separated from his usual living environment and goes into some wild, natural place for a 'vision quest'. Telling good, strong stories at the right moment and in the right place has a powerful effect. There are many youth camps, but few that use the power of mythology effectively. These stories with ancient wisdom and healing are there, waiting to be told.

The heroine's journey

The most popular stories over the past decade or so that I have heard women tell are 'Inanna', 'Skeleton Woman', and 'Vasilisa the Wise'. The latter two stories are to be found in Clarissa Pinkola Estes' *Women Who Run With the Wolves*. All these stories have a strong archetypal death persona at their centre.

'Inanna' is the ancient Sumerian myth, akin to the Greek 'Persephone'. Inanna is queen of heaven and earth and has as her consort Damuzi, the shepherd. Inanna hears the heart-wrenching cries of her sister Ereshkigal grieving over the death of her husband. To meet her sister, she must descend to the lower world of death and no return by passing through seven gates and removing a piece of clothing at each portal. When finally Ereshkigal drains Inanna dry and hangs her lifeless on a hook, life in the upper world dwindles and dies, bringing a winter. The faithful Ninshuba, Inanna's handmaiden, gathers helpers to bring the water of life to Inanna's body. Inanna can return to the upper world if someone will take her place in the depths of the underworld. Demuzi is found sitting on Inanna's throne, and unlike her maidservant and children, does not come to greet her on her return. Demuzi is sent to the underworld to replace Inanna, but his sister Geshtinanna pleads to relieve him of this for half the year. So Demuzi the shepherd 'dies' for half the year, and returns for the other half with his gifts of animal life and fertility.

It is the descent that is so interesting: we have seven layers of skin and seven chakras, or energy points, in our bodies. The image allows us to consider descending into the self, stripping off the outer layers, becoming naked as we face our dark sister, the queen of the underworld. What fears and unknowns are there waiting for us? Going down into the dark areas of oneself is healing and transforming. This ancient story lends itself to be used in a healing ceremony. Women who have used this story report that they can embrace lost parts of themselves as they descend the steps to the underworld. They unearth negative self-beliefs, such as being unlovable, powerless, frozen by fear or rage; with guidance and help they can return up the steps with positive affirmations, bringing back to life their female power, potency and happiness.

'Skeleton Woman' is an extraordinary Inuit story of death and bones lying on the seabed, until the skeleton is fished out from the sea by a lonely fisherman and re-fleshed. Clarissa Pinkola Estes has written a version of the tale based on a five-line poem recited to her by an Inuit woman.

A girl who has done something wrong in her father's eyes is thrown over a cliff into the sea below. There her skeleton is picked clean and lies at the bottom of a cove. Fishermen shun that place, but one night a lonely fisherman finds his boat in the cove, strikes his fishing line into the water, and his hook is caught by something big. Hoping for a big catch, he pulls in something terrifying: skeleton woman. The man steers his boat towards home, but the skeleton holds fast to his boat. Once he lands ashore, the boney bundle clacks and rattles after him, until he reaches his ice-built home. Once inside he lights his lamp and sees that the skeleton has followed him right into his igloo. Compassion for the skeleton makes him untangle the woman from his fishing line and wrap her in furs. When he falls asleep, a tear falls from his eye and skeleton woman drinks this long draught before reaching into the sleeping man and borrowing his heart. She now sings herself some skin, flesh, hair, eyes, and everything she needs to be woman. She returns the heart to the sleeping man and curls up next to him. They wake as a couple.

Estes follows her telling of the story with analysis for creating enduring love by inviting skeleton woman into your life. The life/death/life aspect of skeleton woman gives the fisherman a mate. In that harsh icy climate, the Inuit culture regards taking a mate as forming a resilient yet magical bond with another, which will deepen through all the struggles and hard work to survive. This coupling is enduring love. It endures because both the man and woman recognise the life/death/life aspect of love: they can give up one feature of their attraction and develop another part of their relationship, discovering and growing together to create a strong resilient bond within which both will find treasure. This is a haunting story and attracts many tellers. It is another fabulous tale of archetypal death, and of how we need her to find more lasting relationships, inside a dominant culture of superficial thrills. Skeleton woman will certainly rattle into many hearts and minds, to remind us that there is nothing of value without death.

'Vasilisa the Wise: The Doll in her Pocket' is strongly reminiscent of 'Cinderella', and one of many Russian stories featuring Baba Yaga, the witch, and Vasilisa. In this story, Vasilisa's mother gives her a doll to keep in her pocket before she dies. When her father remarries, Vasilisa is subjected to the scorn of her stepmother and two stepsisters. They plot to get rid of her, and put out the fire and candles so they can demand that Vasilisa go out that very night to fetch fire from Baba Yaga. Vasilisa takes her doll with her, who encourages her and shows her the way through the dark forest. Horses with riders pass her as she journeys: a white one at dawn, a red one at sunrise and a black one at nightfall. Arriving at Baba Yaga's hut in the woods, she asks for fire and is given several tasks to complete in return: cooking for Baba Yaga, washing her clothes, cleaning her house, then sorting the mouldy corn from the good and separating small stones from poppy seeds. She can only complete these arduous, time-consuming tasks with the help of the doll in her pocket, while she herself sleeps. Baba Yaga flies off each night, and on her return summons some mysterious hands to grind the corn and press the seed for oil for her. Baba Yaga is impressed by Vasilisa's skill and, being the keeper of fire, gives her a skull on a stick from her fence. Vasilisa hurries home with the fire in the skull. Her stepmother and sisters have assumed she has been eaten up by Baba Yaga. When they see the light shining from the skull, the 'eyes' seem to follow them, until they burn up and disintegrate into ashes.

This is a strong female initiation story, moving the initiate from powerlessness to the fire of rightful action. Not all versions of this story include a doll in Vasalisa's pocket; I think the story is stronger and clearer with the doll. The doll symbolises intuition or soul guidance and shows that the difficult tasks of cleaning and sorting are best done with help from this aspect of the psyche. The story warns us that being too nice is not good and that a deep wild instinct is required to recognise that most things are not as they seem. The key tasks given to Vasilisa are sorting good corn from mouldy, and stones and dirt from poppy seeds. 'The fresh corn, mildewed corn, poppy seeds and dirt are all remnants of an ancient healing apothecary. These substances are used as salves, balms and poultices to hold other medicines on the body,' says Estes. Here we have evidence that Baba Yaga was an ancient healer using herbal medicines. But she is fierce, and will only give you the plain truth, and maybe eat you up if you stay too long or ask too many questions. She is archetypal as well as practical. This fairy tale has come from an ancient healing wisdom. Because it is a Cinderella-type story, it is very accessible to a wide age range. I have told it dressed simply to young children, and dressed more fully to adults.

Returning women to their wild power, *Women Who Run with the Wolves* (Estes, 1992) presents a woman's journey, giving a story for each aspect of a woman's psyche, complimented by extensive Jungian analysis to many character responses. Powerful and untamed, this book has profound treasures drawn up from a deep well for women to taste; you must dip into its wild waters to see if it is for you. Writing in such intimate detail about the ways women think and feel is revolutionary. Verifying the feelings women have silently and secretly, often alone, this book now brings them into general view, enticing public acceptance.

In recent years there has been great interest in goddess images and stories. There are cards that give images and a short description of each figure's qualities, which can be used to inspire and stimulate those qualities and moods in a woman. This is feminine hunger surfacing in otherwise sterile situations, where there is little room to display and express the pools, lakes and oceans of emotion. The need for stories for children and families is recognised, but the longing of women, girls and mothers to hear the legacy left by ancient women is in the eyes of those who come and hear stories. They gasp in disbelief as they discover a place that they only dreamt of before.

At the age of thirty, I myself went through a significant initiation of life experience, and this enabled me to discover my warrior self. I did the warrior asanas in yoga, learnt how to do simple repairs to my own car, became self-employed, bought a small terraced house and was fiercely proud of my self-reliance. Years later, when stories had fully entered my life, I came across a short story about Rangada, an Indian warrior woman mentioned in the *Mahabharata* and in *Ancient Mirrors of Womanhood* by Merlin Stone. I was able to put many feelings of discovering my warrior woman into this story, balancing it with femininity, the need for women friends, and the precarious way into a man's heart.

Rangada

Arjuna was a great archer and warrior. After his training as a marksman, his teachers told him that to complete his training in leadership he should go on a retreat for one year, to meditate on the qualities needed in a great warrior. During this time he was to live a simple life and take a vow of celibacy. Taking just the necessities for his journey, he rode north into the Himalayan foothills. When he had passed all the villages, he came to a wild forest and a clear rushing river. When he found a clearing beside the water, he felt this was the perfect place for his retreat. He pitched his tent, washed in the river, rolled out his prayer mat in front of his tent, and willingly began to meditate.

Unknown to Arjuna, there was a village deep inside the forest. There, Rangada, an archer and warrior herself, was held in great respect. If the men needed to ward off thieves and invaders, Rangada would ride out in front. Her youth, beauty and fearlessness gave them courage.

One day she hunted and brought down a deer, skinned it and divided up the meat for the village. Dirty and bloodstained she went to the river to wash. As she came out of the trees she saw a man sitting deep in meditation. He was not like her village men, but calm, perfectly formed, yet utterly powerful. She was spellbound by him, finding deep passions arising within herself. Hearing someone approach, Arjuna broke his meditation to look at his visitor. Forgetting that she was covered in dirt and animal blood, and being accustomed to speaking her mind, she began to tell Arjuna how she felt about him. He silenced her:

'I have taken a vow of celibacy, and besides you are not my idea of womanhood. Leave me in peace!'

Rangada withdrew back to her village. Her womenfolk made her a warm bath scented with cleansing forest herbs. They massaged her tired limbs, washed and oiled her body, combed out her hair and soothed her bruised heart. They brought her ceremonial silk sari and dressed her in it. They put jewels in her hair and bracelets on her wrists and ankles. When she was ready, she walked once again to the clearing beside the river. Slowly and silently she picked her way towards Arjuna, now deep in meditation inside his tent. She lay down on his mat in front of him and waited.

Many minutes went by till Arjuna reached for his bell to complete his practice. His eyes fell upon a most perfect form of womanhood. Had his meditation been so deep that he had conjured up this perfect form? He took the woman by the hand, and they wandered the riverbank, gazing into each other's eyes. She said her name was Malha. As evening became dusk, Arjuna took her into his tent, and broke his vow of celibacy again and again and again! The lovers remained together for the following twelve months.

Back in Rangada's village, her menfolk were looking for her. Several cattle had been stolen and homes invaded by the young men in the next village. It was time to go and face the intruders. They went to the riverside clearing and called for her. Arjuna was sitting outside his tent.

'Have you seen Rangada, our warrior woman?' they asked. 'We need her to ride out with us to defend our village.' Arjuna thought for a moment.

'I saw a woman some months ago, when she came to the river, but not since then.'

'You could not mistake Rangada,' the men said. 'She is not only beautiful, but a skilled archer, horsewoman and as fearless as a lion.'

Inside the tent, Rangada heard the pleading voices of her menfolk. She emerged to speak to them. Arjuna watched, astonished and amazed, as the men were overjoyed to see his gentle 'Mahla', throwing themselves at her feet.

'I am an archer and a warrior. I will ride out with you too,' he offered. They saddled up their horses, took their spears and rode out together, with Rangada at the head. As they rode, Arjuna looked at Rangada – her muscles easily held her horse, sweat stood on her skin and her hair flew wildly behind her – and loved her for the warrior woman she was.

What do we mean by our 'journey of life'? What can we hope to achieve in our lives? Perhaps a maturity, so we can be effective in the present society; perhaps an unfolding of our skills, abilities and intuitions – an awakening; perhaps the healing of past traumas for ourselves and relatives. I have no recipe, but I do have the scent of my own pathway in my responses to a powerful story. It is the quickening of my blood, the need to breathe deeper, the desire to mull over certain key phrases or characters. For me this usually means I need to tell the story many times to sift and pan its rivers and sources. Once we have taken the stopper out of the genie's bottle, we cannot control the powers. I believe the same is true for stories: a story must be set free to work its magic, and can never be definitively prescribed for a particular task. Its effect depends on who hears it.

The King Who was Miserable

There was once a king who was miserable. If he was presented with a perfectly ripe peach for his breakfast, he would find a worm in it. If he ordered a soft pear for his elevenses, he would find it was bruised and rotting at its centre. If he wore his cotton shirt, the seams would chaff him; when he put on his silk shirt, it would be too soft, too slippery. Nothing pleased him. He thought about this, and as he looked out of his window, he saw the very ordinary people in the market within the great city walls, buying and selling and going about their business. He thought, 'There must be some very poor wretch in my city that, through poverty and hard work, is more miserable than I.'

That evening, which happened to be a Friday, without telling anyone but his closest servant, he changed his royal robes for those of an ordinary working person and stepped out into the twilight air of the streets. He wandered, looking and listening, into the shanty town that had sprung up just outside the city walls. He came to a very home-made, ramshackle hut, its door hanging askew on its hinges. Surely there must be a very wretched person living here, he thought.

Approaching the door, with his hand ready to knock, he heard singing coming from inside,

'Shabbat shalom, Shabbat shalom, Shabbat, Shabbat, Shabbat, Shabbat shalom...'

The disguised king's shadow announced his presence, the door opened, and a lean, tanned but smiling face greeted him,

'My friend, you have come on the Sabbath evening, and this is twice the reason to celebrate! Come in, and let the feast begin!'

The king entered the shabby hut and sat on old stool. The 'feast' before him was merely sweet Jewish bread – challah – and water. But the ordinary man sang more songs, cracked jokes, divided the fresh bread, and the two ate it up. He was a shoeshine man, he said, and today he was happy he had earned enough to celebrate the eve of the holy day of Saturday. The King ate and listened.

He returned to his palace, peeved. How could this shoeshine man, who lived in a shack, be so very happy? Maybe he was not poor enough. By morning the king had formed a plan. He decreed that all shoeshine workers were banned from plying their trade within the city walls. Everyone knew that if you could not work within the city's market streets, there was little chance of getting customers.

The following Friday evening, the king, wearing his disguise, made his way into the shanty town and knocked at the ordinary man's door. Now, thought the king, I will see if he still has a smile on his face! The door opened, and there was the lean but smiling face, welcoming him inside. He related to the king, that shoeshinning had been banished, so he had exchanged his brushes and polish for a water jar, and had spent the week selling water inside the city. How lucrative that had been!

'Here I have fish, bread and wine to offer to you today, my friend!' With that, he began to sing, 'Lai la lai la, lai la lai la...'

The king found himself joining in.

The next morning the king decreed all water sellers were banned from the city market places.

'This should test the smile on his face,' thought the king, wringing his hands together.

Friday evening came, and the king, in disguise once again, knocked at the ordinary man's door. He was welcomed by a lean and even more smiling face,

'Ah, my friend, we can celebrate the Sabbath in style tonight! When water sellers were banned, I was lucky enough to exchange my urn for a good axe. This week I have sold firewood in the city, and have earned good money. See, here, the feast I can offer you.' The ordinary man sat the king beside a table laid with bread, fish, fruit, cakes and wine. He was so merry, even the king began to smile.

When the king returned to the palace, he resolved to find another way. The next morning he announced that all firewood sellers would be conscripted into the army. The ordinary man found himself marching up and down the royal courtyard, with a new uniform, boots and a steel sword at his side. At the end of the first week, he went to his commanding officer and asked him for his weekly wage. He was dismayed when he received the reply that he would be paid a salary at the end of each month. 'How can I celebrate the Sabbath tonight?' he thought. He looked at the fine new sword at his side, and went off to the pawnbrokers. Late that afternoon, he got two pieces of wood and fashioned them into a sword which fitted into the sheath. That evening, the king heard from the ordinary man how he had pawned his sword. It did not take the king long before he had hatched the perfect plan to catch out this persistently happy and resourceful man.

The next morning, with great satisfaction, the king summoned his troops into the royal courtyard.

'In the name of justice, here is a young boy who has stolen a melon from the royal gardens.' A young boy was brought forward, head hung low. 'This is an offence punishable by death. I would like one of my soldiers to execute him. You there, step forward.' The king pointed to the ordinary shoeshine man, knowing that he did not have his sword, and so would be severely punished. The ordinary man stepped forward, and faced the crowd, pausing to say his prayers and asking for help.

'I pray to the great one, whose name cannot be mentioned, that if this young man should be pardoned for his youthful folly, my sword be turned to wood!' He took out his sword with a flourish, so all could see that it was made of wood.

A gasp of wonder went around the crowd, then a hushed silence. As all these people had witnessed the divine transformation, the king was compelled to grant a pardon to the boy, and set him free.

While the crowd dispersed, the king felt a strange tickle in his belly which grew and grew, rising up to his throat, and out through his mouth as loud bellowing laughter. He laughed and laughed, as he had never laughed before. Then he sent for that soldier who was the ordinary shoeshine man, and invited him to become his first minister. The king spent many hours a week with his new minister, asking his advice on all court matters.

Years went by, and whether the king took the Jewish faith or not is not known. But from then on, the king was seen to smile. The king and his first minister grew old together, and they died in the same year, in the same month, on the same day, with the same breath.

I doubt whether two people reading this story would agree to its meaning. However, the ordinary but happy man is flexible, resourceful, and changes as needs arise in order to survive, and this does not diminish his happiness, but increases it. The miserable king pursues the happy man relentlessly, beyond normal interest. Of course, we realise he wants to know how such a poor man *can* be so happy; the ending of the story confirms that he wanted to become like the happy man. A king is a person who has a lot of power and choice; there is a spark in this king that seeks happiness even if he has to search outside his usual circles, going on an adventure into places he has rarely if ever been before. This demonstrates to the listener of the story the force from within that cannot be denied. A wealthy and privileged man must change his clothes and be as an ordinary one in order to discover what will satisfy his inner craving.

To me, this old story shows very clearly and with great wit, the power of the inner human drive for growth. Meeting challenges on the way through life and being able to change outwardly, while inwardly keeping alive the same qualities, or faith, brings great satisfaction and happiness. My interest in this story shows this is something I am facing in my own life.

There is a growing awareness that we are nature, and not separate beings somehow divinely privileged, as some Christian texts would have us believe. We breathe air cleaned by trees and plants, we eat food grown on our planet: there is some large part of ourselves that must obey the laws of the living earth. We are seeds, we sprout and, tended with water, food and loving care, we grow to flower and fruit, until ripe enough to let our seeds drop to the earth.

Our developing consciousness, backed up with our phenomenal communication skills of speech, reading and writing has given us a sense of superior divine blessing. Logical thinking about our dependence on the whole web of life on earth signifies to me that everything is linked; if one life form is sacred, so are all the interwoven life forms. We can no longer separate ourselves as specially conscious and therefore the only animal divinely connected to a creator, the one who guides us on our path through life, to attain great insights and achievements. That idea is from a past time, a way to help people realise their power of consciousness. Everything must grow and change, including religious beliefs and attitudes. We want to find the eternal truths, to feel the security and comfort of them around us. But walking up the eternal mountain of life, at every peak we see there is yet more to climb. When we can bear the insecurity, we may be able to trust the present moment of our existence, as it continues to change.

The gift of story can help us by connecting us to our past and providing imaginative tools to create the future.

9. An exercise of the spirit

There is a dream dreaming us.

SAYING OF THE KALAHARI BUSHMAN

Evolution is not just something that happened to the dinosaurs, or when the first life forms crept out of the oceans: evolution is ongoing. It seems as if all life forms, including humans, have reached the peak of their physical development, so is there something else that evolution is working on? Some sceptics say this is an age of self-indulgence. In my experience, what is happening now is all for a purpose, to prepare for the next stage, and to deny it will only delay its effectiveness.

In 1990 I worked as an English language teacher in Brunei, Borneo, a small country bordered by Malaysia and Kalimantan. Thinking of new ways to interest the children, I chose a rhythmic, rhyming poem and asked one child to read the first line. He refused by folding his arms and looking determinedly offended. Yet when I tried asking the whole front row to read the first line out aloud, they willingly and easily did this. The children were between nine and eleven years old, but they could not separate themselves from their peers. At this point in their educational development, which involved a culture of chanting and ceremony for every occasion, collective progress was encouraged. I realised that the children had a kind of group consciousness, in contrast to my British training, which focused on individual achievement.

When I reflected on my own upbringing, I saw that I myself had been through a phase of not seeing myself as separate from my family. I did not question my inherited family ways and values until I met non-family members, until life forced me to question and change those habitual ways of talking and relating as if everyone around me would understand what I meant. I was forced to recognise other people behaving in their individual ways, and this developed my own unique identity. I see this as evidence of a group identity gradually evolving to become a more individual one. We can all look back to the lives of our grandparents and be aware of the changes in thinking, attitude and lifestyle. These changes carry evolution at work, even if we do not like it, even if it does not appear healthy, it is still change going somewhere, which will motivate further change, and be adapted later on. The wise invisible friend who resides in the deep psyche of us all makes sure that progress is made in human development, whether we are conscious of it or not.

What are the changes going on at this time where you are? Where I am, people are concerned with 'self development' in most walks of life. In industry, managers are undergoing training courses to help them cope with their job of sustaining a satisfied and cohesive workforce. Head teachers are required to understand group dynamics and find ways to listen to 'difficult' parents and children. Couples want to relate to each other in ever more satisfying ways. Seekers are able to choose what path to explore in the profusion of Buddhist and meditation centres of many kinds. Yoga arrived in public view in the UK in the sixties, with the Beatles giving it pop culture approval; now, it can be found in every town, village and community hall. In forty years it has shifted from an unknown, radical activity to a mainstream one. Psychotherapy, drama therapy, psychodynamic counselling, and so many more therapies are in full flood, advertised in magazines, at 'mind, body, spirit' festivals, and probably in your local shop window too. This has developed over the past two decades.

We want to grow, progress and be healed in order to fulfil our lives. We need guidelines and prompts along the way. Story gives us the feast from which we can forage and taste good food as we travel through life's prickly forests, bleak deserts, remote islands and dark tunnels.

Jumping Mouse

Once, in the roots of an old tree, there lived a family of mice. They moved seeds from here to there and there to here. They were busy and their whiskers twitched constantly. But there was one mouse who one day stopped and listened. He heard a roaring sound in his ears. He went to his brother.

'Can you hear a roaring sound in your ears?' he asked.

'No, I can't. We're busy. Come on, help move these seeds,' came the reply.

And he got the same reply from all his other brothers and sisters. He felt very alone. So one day he began the journey towards that roaring sound, leaving the safety of the roots of the old tree. As he scurried along, he looked about him. He saw things he'd never seen before: flowers, butterflies, birds, insects and the sunlight that flickered through the leaves. He was happy. Then he heard a voice.

'Brother mouse, you are far from home, what are you doing here?' It was brother racoon sitting in the branches of a tree.

'Brother racoon, I can hear a roaring sound in my ears, and I want to know what it is,' called out the mouse.

'Oh yes, the roaring sound. Why, that is the great river, the great river of life. I am coming down myself, to wash these berries. I'll show you where it is,' came the reply.

The little mouse was amazed. There really was something that made the roaring sound? He followed brother racoon down the path and soon they came out of the undergrowth. Then he saw it. Roaring, rushing water, sparkling in the sunlight. Brother racoon washed his berries in the water.

'Let me introduce you to a friend of mine.' He took the little mouse to a lily pad where a green frog was resting half in and half out of the water. 'This is brother frog. Now I must leave you, brother mouse.'

The mouse thanked brother racoon, and lingered by that rushing river.

'Brother mouse, would you like some medicine?' asked brother frog. The little mouse had no idea what medicine was, but everything was new and exciting that day.

'Yes, yes, I'd like some medicine,' he said.

'Well then, crouch down as low as you can and jump up as high as you can,' said the frog.

The little mouse crouched down as low as he could and leapt up as high as he could. He saw over the great river, over the hot plain, he saw far away in the distance the high peaks of the sacred mountains. But now something else was happening, he was beginning to fall down. He fell with a splash into the water. Luckily the river was quite shallow there and he quickly scrambled out onto the bank.

'You've tricked me, I'm wet and cold,' said the mouse.

'But you're not hurt, are you?' said brother frog. 'Do not let your fear and anger blind you. Did you see something?'

'I saw the sacred mountains,' said brother mouse.

'Well then, you got your medicine. And you've got a new name: it is Jumping Mouse.'

'Jumping Mouse,' thought the little mouse.

Now he wanted to return home to tell his brothers and sisters. He thanked brother frog and, keeping the roaring sound at his back, he hurried home along the path. Leaves and small twigs stuck to his wet fur as he went. When he got to the roots of the old tree his brothers and sisters shook their heads.

'He must have been caught in the jaws of some great animal and spat out,' they whispered, 'he's probably poisonous.' They shrank away from him, and wouldn't speak to him.

Jumping Mouse felt even lonelier than before. He

rested, dried and cleaned his fur, ate some seeds and tried to live as other mice did. But before long he felt so restless that he realised what he would have to do. He turned his back on the safety of life in the roots of the old tree, and set out again towards the roaring sound, determined to find the sacred mountains. When he came to the great river, he followed it till he came to the edge of the hot plain. He looked up in the sky and saw many black spots wheeling overhead. Every mouse knows the black spots are eagles that swoop down and eat you up should you run out into the open. He came to a sweet sage patch and thankfully crept inside. Then he heard another voice,

'Welcome, brother mouse, you are welcome to share my home.' It was an old, old mouse. They ate together and exchanged their news. But when he heard that Jumping Mouse wanted to go to the sacred mountains, the old mouse explained,

'The great river exists, but the sacred mountains, they are just a myth. You better stay here with me. We have journeyed further than any mice before us. The black spots will surely get you if you attempt to cross the plain.' Jumping Mouse now knew he would have to continue his journey to the sacred mountains alone.

Next morning he ran out of the sweet sage patch and stumbled into a mound covered with fur and black horns. He heard a groaning sound coming from it.

'I am sick, and my medicine tells me that only the eye of a mouse can save me. But mice do not exist, so I shall die.' It was a buffalo lying with its head on the ground. 'I am a mouse and this is a great beast, far greater than I,' thought Jumping Mouse. He paused for a moment, then went up to the buffalo.

'Brother Buffalo, you are a greater being than I, if one of my eyes can save you, you can have it.'

Immediately he said this, one of his eyes flew out of his

head into the buffalo. The buffalo got to his feet, completely healed,

'Brother Jumping Mouse, you are a great brother, for you have made me whole. I know of your quest to go to the sacred mountains. I will take you across the plain. Walk between my hooves, under the shelter of my body.' Jumping Mouse ran as fast as he could to keep up with the buffalo. The sound of the buffalo's hooves was deafening, and with only one eye the little mouse was frightened he would be trampled on. At last they reached the edge of the plain, at the foot of the sacred mountains. 'Brother Jumping Mouse, this is as far as I can take you. But if ever you need me, you know where to find me,' said the buffalo, as he turned to go back across the plain.

Jumping Mouse looked up. The sacred mountains were still a long way away, and he could see black spots overhead. He ran into the shade of a rock, when he heard another strange voice.

'I've eaten what I've forgotten and I've forgotten what I've eaten. Am I a wolf or am I not?' He looked around and saw a wolf chasing its own tail round and round. 'This is a being greater than I. It has lost its memory, and I think I know how to heal it,' thought Jumping Mouse. He went up to the wolf,

'Brother Wolf, you are a greater being than I am, and if one of my eyes can heal you, you can have it.' Immediately he said this, his other eye flew from his head into the body of the wolf. The wolf regained his memory and as he looked down at the little mouse, a tear came to his eye. But Jumping Mouse could not see this, as he was now completely blind.

'Brother Jumping Mouse, you are indeed a great brother for you have made me whole. I will take you up the sacred mountain to the great medicine lake. Climb up on my back,' said the wolf. Feeling the warmth of the wolf, the little mouse edged forward and climbed onto its back. Up and up a zigzag path they went. Jumping Mouse could feel the cool air on his face as they climbed higher. Finally they arrived at the great medicine lake. Jumping Mouse got down from the wolf's back and asked the wolf to describe the place to him. He crawled to the edge of the lake for a cool, refreshing drink.

'Brother Jumping Mouse, I must leave you now, but if ever you need me, you know where to find me,' said the wolf as he turned to go back down the mountain.

Jumping Mouse knew there was now no shelter from the black spots. Soon he heard the sound that eagles make, and felt the wind from powerful wings above him. Then the claws struck on his back, and he fell asleep. When he awoke, he opened his eyes and he could see, though blurrily at first. He heard a familiar voice,

'Brother Jumping Mouse, would you like some medicine?'

'Oh yes, yes,' replied Jumping Mouse.

'Then crouch down as low as you can, and jump up as high as you can.' He crouched down as low as he could and leapt up as high as he could. He began to see more clearly than before, and he saw brother frog beside the medicine lake.

'Lean into the wind and trust,' said brother frog. Jumping Mouse felt he had wings, a tail and a beak and he was flying higher and higher. 'Brother Jumping Mouse, you now have a new name: it is Eagle.'

Soaring higher, he spread his wings, gliding over the sacred mountains and down towards the plain. He saw brother wolf, brother buffalo and brother racoon. They all looked up and called out,

'Hello Brother Eagle!'

This is a sacred teaching story from Indigenous American tradition, which has been generously written down to share. Please treat it with respect by giving thanks to the old tellers who have lovingly kept it alive and, if you are familiar with such ceremonies, offer tobacco or chocolate in gratitude. The original written story and the intention behind this beautiful teaching story can be found in *Seven Arrows* by Hyemeyohsts Storm, given as part of the Sun Dance way.

I was lucky enough to hear 'Jumping Mouse' told by storyteller Tim Bowley round a fire in a field full of tents, where it flowed and mused with feathers of its own. Some storytellers think it is a children's story, others an adult one. The story is extraordinary for European ears, with its clear insight into the human journey told through animal eyes. Giving up our way of seeing as a mouse to gain an eagle's ultimate clarity of vision! 'Don't let your fear and anger blind you,' warns the frog. Jumping Mouse finds an old mouse in a sage patch, but the old mouse cannot see the sacred mountains from the security of his 'sage' or wisdom: 'the black spots will get you if you go further,' he warns the young mouse. But Jumping Mouse has seen the sacred mountains, and knows he must face the fear of being devoured. It is not learnt wisdom that takes us there, but going out into everyday life, trusting to our heartfelt feeling and intuition of the right way.

The Secret of Creation

The Great Creator had finished making the sun, the earth, the moon and the stars. On the earth he had completed the forests, seas, plants and trees, animals and birds, and finally the human beings. As the humans breathed and moved about, the Creator saw that sometimes they were sad as well as happy. Sometimes they felt alone and bewildered as well as contented. The Creator decided he would put the answer to these feelings in a secret that he would hide in a place they would have to search for.

He summoned all the animals together and asked them where the best place would be to hide this secret.

The whale came forward, 'I can swim to the depths of the seas, and hide it there.'

'Ah, the humans are very clever, and will find a way of delving into even the deepest oceans. They will easily find it there,' replied the Creator.

The eagle swooped down, 'I can fly to the top of the highest snow-capped mountains and hide it there.'

'The humans are clever enough to go to the top of the highest mountain, they will find it there,' said the Creator.

The stag leapt up, 'I can go into the deepest forest and hide it there.'

'Oh, I'm afraid the humans are clever enough to find it there,' said the Creator.

Then the earth beneath them began to move, and they all stood back. Soon a small quivering nose and two powerful yet small clawed hands appeared above the ground. It was mole.

'I have been listening to what you have said, and I know a place the humans will never find the secret.'

The Creator looked down at mole. 'Tell us where that is.'

'Well, if you hide the secret of their creation deep inside their own hearts, they will never think of looking there!'

The Creator addressed all the animals,

'You are right, mole, the humans are clever enough to explore all of the earth, but the last place they will look is inside their own hearts!'

This story probably originates from India, where Brahman wants to find a hiding place for the divinity of the gods who abused their power and were made into humans. (See 'Where Could One Hide It' in the Bibliography.) This version is told in the Native

American Indian or First Nation style.

The mystical element of stories

'Enchantment is our natural state,' writes Deepak Chopra (Chopra, 1994), meaning that the source of all our thoughts, health, actions and entire being begin with connection to the cosmic energies of life itself! However, if we are not able to grasp this, all we need to do is acknowledge the feeling of enchantment within ourselves. We call it dreaming, being lost in thought or what we are doing, day dreaming, wonder or enchantment. It is seen very clearly in children, and it is captivating to adults. Gazing at a baby, adults can experience the enchantment of the fresh, newly arrived person in its pure expression. It is this enchantment that stories told well and appropriately can arouse and touch. Children need to experience it often to feel its nourishment. The benefits of storytelling to children cannot be easily verified, as stories can be stored up in their consciousness as wisdom for a later time; this is their 'magic'. At the present time in schools, activities are being considered for their usefulness in child development according to their practical outcome or supposed benefit. But storytelling, by its magical nature, cannot be assessed in this way. It may be used to introduce topics and capture children's interest and attention, but the medicine of a story is as free as air. Teachers know in their hearts that learning is not linear and that they are called to respond to the needs of children, by listening to them. Experienced teachers know that example speaks louder than words, that respect and trust is earnt by the way they treat the children. And, most of all, to expect the unexpected, to be able to 'think on their feet' to meet what the children cry out for. The unquantifiable, the mystical and magical element is always there. Stories need to be set free to work their magic.

Healing time

> On a personal level, we are being asked to clean up and heal our thoughts, our emotions, our intentions, our old pain, our denials, our physical health and our actions. When we become personally responsible for the healing of every thought, action, intention and deed in our lives, the rest of the world will heal along with us. (Sams, 1994)

We may have lost our ancient 'blood' or connection with life forces, but with our newly developed consciousness and reason, there are signs that we are now able to bring holistic feeling and thinking into our lives. I feel this when I tell a story to responsive audience. We communicate many things beyond reason and the flow of words, which satisfies soul longing.

There are archetypes living in each of us, and it is possible that on some level we can respond to the ancient picture language of the old storytellers. One of the tasks of the contemporary storyteller is to bring ancient stories to modern ears, using the teller–listener connection to create a bridge on which wisdom and healing can take place. Opening our imaginations, with purposeful intention and careful intuition, we can co-create a future full of the best of human values.

Responsibility for intention and speech

We can be very creative with our speech in conversations. On a November day, I could say, 'It's cold, misty and dreary today!' Another way to express the weather could be, 'Autumn has enveloped us in its mists and mellow fruitfulness.' One has negative feelings in it, the other, joyful ones, yet they describe the same weather. Our intention and feelings are expressed in the words we choose.

129

If we become 'mindful', that is, aware of what we are offering another person in a conversation, we may wish to modify or change how we are communicating. Consider the concern that many small shops have closed because of the recession. If I am someone with a good business head, then I could say, 'What an opportunity to start a good business; I can see what is needed here.' The limitation is our own.

Unchallenged complaint and limitations can start a negative culture. 'There is so much violence on TV and in the news, I no longer feel safe to go out.' This is quite often said and heard in the UK. There is some truth in it: there is violence on TV and the news. But it is safer to go on a journey now than it ever has been in past history. In Elizabethan times, robbery and mugging were commonplace; if you had not taken to the new Church of England but were still a practising Catholic you might also have a price on your head. The violent programmes on TV and radio can be switched off and we can choose not to be so focussed on that view of life. The media has a reputation for over-dramatising events in order to sell newspapers and get high ratings for programmes. Going out into the streets in unknown districts should certainly be done with good sense, and with reliable, firsthand information taken into account, but media hype should not deter us from making the journey. The media's interest in violence, wars and death has become a mantra of fear and injury recited to the nation every day. I inherited some tape recordings of music concerts on the radio. But my stepfather also recorded the news at the end of the concerts. I drive along in my car listening to fine music, then comes the news in usual format: war in another country, acts of violence to people, protests, fraud uncovered, arrests by police, appearances in court and so on. Suddenly the tape ends and I realise I have been listening to news over fifteen years old! It sounds almost the same as contemporary news.

The way we communicate with each other helps form a new reality. The words we use and the intention behind them are given to others as conversational stories. By repeating negative clichés we keep each other trapped in pervading attitudes. We are in a fear culture at present, because we are becoming more aware, we meet a greater variety of people than we did in the past, we work in many different and ever-changing ways as we try to keep up with technology and social change and the rapid rise in global population. Our consciousness has changed. We need new skills to cope creatively with these changes. Positive thinking and mindfulness can lead to open-minded progress with contemporary challenges, where we offer each other fresh, thoughtful, positive conversation. This is, then, good ground, in which co-creating a wonderful future can take place from our higher nature.

Bibliography

Avery, Gillian (1995) *Russian Fairy Tales* Everyman Library.

Bettelheim, Bruno (1991) *The Uses of Enchantment,* Penguin Books.

Bly, Robert (1991) *Iron John,* Element Books.

Bolen, Jean Shinoda (2001) *Goddesses in Older Women*, Harper Collins.

Campbell, Joseph (1993) *The Hero with a Thousand Faces,* Fontana Press.

Carey, D. and J. Large (1982) *Festivals, Family and Food*, Hawthorn Press.

Carter, Angela (1991) *The Virago Book of Fairy Tales*, Virago Press.

Childs, Gilbert (1993) *Steiner Education,* Floris Books.

Chodzin, S. and Kohn, A. (1997) *Buddhist Tales*, Barefoot Books.

Chopra, Deepak (1994) *Journey into Healing,* Rider.

Chrispeels and Colebrook (2003) *The Triple Mirror*, Green Spirit.

Colum, Padraic (1994) *King of Ireland's Son,* Floris Books.

Colum, Padraic (1983) Introduction, *The Complete Grimm*, Routledge.

Corrin, S. and S. (1988) in *The Faber Book of Favourite Fairy Tales*, Guild Publishing.

Diop, Birago (1985) *Tales of Amadou Koumba*, Longman African Classics.

Dwivedi, K.N. (1997) in *The Therapeutic Use of Stories,* by Damian Gardner, Routledge.

Eschenbach, Wolfram von (1980) *Parsifal*, trans. A.T. Hatto, Penguin Classics.

Estes, Clarissa Pinkola (1992) *Women Who Run With the Wolves*, Random House.

Feldman,C. And Kornfield J. (1991) *Stories of the Spirit, Stories of the Heart,* Harper Collins.

Fitzjohn,Weston and Large (2001) *Festivals Together,* Hawthorn Press.

Gersie, A. (1992) *Earthtales: Storytelling in Times of Change,* Green Print.

Gwyndaf, Robin (1989) *Welsh Folk Tales*, National Museum of Wales.

Hall, Kelvin (2000) *Beyond the Forest,* Hawthorn Press.

Hayes, B., Lodge, M., Ingpen, R. (1992) *Folk Tales and Fables of the Middle East and Africa*, Dragon's World.

Hennessey, Nick (2001) compact disk *Of Fire, Wind and Silver Stream*.

Jones, Gwyn and Thomas (1984) *Mabinogion*, Everyman's Library.

Knijpenga, Siegwart (1997) *Stories of the Saints*, Floris Books.

Kumar, Satish (2004) *The Buddha and the Terrorist,* Green Books.

Lancelyn Green, Roger (1993) *King Arthur and his Knights,* Everyman's Library.

Lancelyn Green, Roger (1995) *The Tales of Greek Heroes,* Puffin Classics.

Lancelyn Green, Roger (2011) *Tales of Ancient Egypt,* Puffin Classics.

Lievegood, Bernard (1997) *Phases of Childhood,* Floris Books.

Maddern, Eric (1993) *Earth Story*, Francis Lincoln.

Matthews, John (1997) *Healing The Wounded King,* Element Books.

Mayo, Margaret (1994) *The Orchard Book of Magical Tales,* Orchard Books.

McCaughrean, Geraldine (1992) *The Orchard Book of Greek Myths,* Orchard Books.

Mellon, Nancy (2000) *Storytelling with Children*, Hawthorn Press.

Mellon, Nancy (1993) *Storytelling and the Art of the Imagination,* Element Books.

Meyer, Rudolf (1988) *The Wisdom of Fairy Tales,* Floris Books.

Milbourne, A. (2004) *Stories from India*, Usborne Publishing.

Naidu, Vayu (1993) 'Ganesha', audio tape, *Katha Yatra.*

Patten, Brian and Mary Moore (2010) *Jumping Mouse*, Hawthorn Press.

Perrow, Susan (2008) *Healing Stories for Challenging Behaviour,* Hawthorn Press.

Sams, Jamie (1994) *Earth Medicine,* Harper Collins.

Shah, Idries (1998) *World Tales,* Octagon Press.

Sheldrake, Rupert (2004) *The Sense of Being Stared At*, Arrow Books.

Sierra, Judy (1992) *Cinderella*, Oryx Press.

Sierra, Judy (1994) *Quests and Spells,* BKMA.

Skynner, R. and Cleese, J. (1983) *Families and How to Survive Them,* Cedar.

Stockmeyer, Karl (1991) *Rudolf Steiner's Curriculum for Waldorf Schools,* Robinswood.

Thomas, T. and Killick, S. (2007) *Telling Tales: Storytelling as Emotional Literacy,* E-Publishing.

Troyes, Chretian de (1976) *Perceval (The Story of the Grail)*, Boydell & Brewer.

Wolkstein, D. (1983) *Innana, Queen of Heaven and Earth,* Harper & Row.

Wood, A. and Richardson R. (1992) *Inside Stories*, Trentham Books.

Story Sources

'Cinderella', 'Iron Hans', 'Rapunzel', 'The Devil with Three Golden Hairs', 'The Frog King', 'The Goose Girl', 'The Juniper Tree' and 'The Two Brothers' *The Complete Grimm's Fairytales* Jacob and Wilhelm Grimm, Routledge, 1993.

'Jumping Mouse' *Seven Arrows* Hyemeyohsts Storm, Ballantine Books, 1972.

'Rangada' *Ancient Mirrors of Womanhood* Merlin Stone, Beacon Press, 1984.

'The Black Prince' audio tape *Making Peace* Laura Simms.

'The Cracked Pot' *Tales from the Tsunami Trail,* Society for Storytelling booklet, 2005.

'The Story of Creation' from 'Where Could one Hide it?' *The Gentle Art of Blessing* Pierre Pradervand, Cygnus Books, 2003.

'The Three Golden Eggs 1 and 2' by the author from a written version, 'The Three Eggs' *Storymaking in Education and Therapy*, Gersie and King, Jessica Kingsley, 1990.

'Tom Who Was Scared of the Dark' audio tape *All Through the Night* Jan Williams, 1994.

'Truth and Story', 'Maybe, Maybe Not', 'The Prince and the Ring', 'A New Dawn', 'The Man who was Sad', 'The Tree at the Crossroads', 'The Hollow in the Stone', 'How an African Hunts', 'The Rabbi's Gift', 'The Listener', 'The King who was Miserable', 'The Secret of Creation' and 'Seventeen Camels' were heard from other storytellers in the aural tradition.

Useful Websites

Society for Storytelling
www.sfs.org.uk
Official site with events diary
of story clubs, storytellers'
directory and *Storylines*
magazine and more.

Story Arts
www.storyarts.org
Encouages storytelling in the
classroom and across the
curriculum with a treasure-chest
of ideas.

Stories for the Seasons
www.h-net.org/~nilas/seasons/
Nature and seasonal stories
for primary children with a
bibliography for stories of
animals and plants.

Storytelling and Arts
Empowerment
www.artslynx.org/heal/stories.
htm
How storytelling and the arts can
build strong individuals and
communities.

Tales of Wonder
www.darsie.net/tales of wonder
An archive of fairy tales and folk
tales from many parts of the
world.

Story Lovers Website
www.story-lovers.com/index.html
Find the world's best-loved stories
and rhymes, their sources,
and advice from professional
storytellers.

Collection of Grimms Tales
www.cs.cmu.edu/-spok/
grimmtmp
Most of the tales of Grimm based
on the translation by Margaret
Hunt.

Indigenous Peoples Literature
www.indigenouspeople.net
Central site for indigenous
literature worldwide.

Kid's Storytelling Club
www.storycraft.com
Resources for young storytellers
with ideas for storytelling aids
and more.

Alliance for Childhood
www.allianceforchildhood.org
A worldwide organisation that
promotes healthy, creative and
joyful education and living.

Emerson College
www.emerson.org.uk
The college offers a three-month
storytelling course each autumn,
and many drama, crafts, voice
and Steiner-Waldorf education
courses.

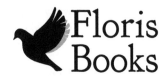

Floris Books

For news on all the latest books, and
exclusive discounts, join our mailing list at:

florisbooks.co.uk/signup

And get a FREE book
with every online order!

We will never pass your details to anyone else.